Invitation to
MEDICINE

Other titles in preparation

Invitation to
MEDICINE

Douglas Black

BASIL BLACKWELL

First published 1987

Basil Blackwell Ltd
108 Cowley Road, Oxford, OX4 1JF, UK

Basil Blackwell Inc.
432 Park Avenue South, Suite 1503
New York, NY 10016, USA

British Library Cataloguing in Publication Data
Black, Sir Douglas
Invitation to medicine. — (Invitations)
1. Medicine — Vocational guidance
I. Title
610.69   R690

ISBN 0-631-14764-0
ISBN 0-631-14765-9 pbk

Library of Congress Cataloging in Publication Data
Black, Douglas, Sir.
Invitation to medicine.
(Invitation series)
Includes index.
1. Medicine. 2. Public health. 3. Medicine —
Vocational guidance. I. Title. II. Series.
[DNLM: 1. Medicine. WB 100 B627i]
R130.B53 1987   610'.69   86-20637
ISBN 0-631-14764-0
ISBN 0-631-14765-9 (pbk.)

Typeset in 10 on 11½pt Bembo
by Columns of Reading
Printed in Great Britain by
Page Bros (Norwich) Ltd

Contents

Contents

Preface

The practice of medicine cannot be learned from books, nor can it even be taught by teachers. It can come in its entirety only from constant and prolonged interchanges with patients. A glance at any of the massive student textbooks of medicine, or at a shelf of monographs dealing with a single system or organ of the body, will show that even the theoretical aspects of medicine could in no way be covered by a book of this size and scope – that is not its purpose. As with other members of the series, its aim is to give some indication of the flavour of medical practice, in all its rich variety, including the care of populations as well as that of individuals. The book may have something to offer the sixth-former considering medicine as a career; the lay person with a general interest in medicine; and even (since the author is primarily a clinician) scientists working on medical problems without themselves being qualified to practise clinical medicine, a group from whom so many valuable contributions have come.

The book divides into three main sections. In the first of these (chapters 1–3), I try to give some inkling of the nature of the scientific knowledge that underpins the practice of medicine. If you look at a textbook of medicine, you will see that it is crammed with facts, but underneath all these are some more general ideas on broad matters such as heredity and environment, the nature of disease processes in general and so on. I have tried to extract these principles, using hard facts as illustrations, and not attempting the impossible task of being comprehensive. Even so, you may find these few chapters heavy going, simply because they are so compressed.

When you have won through these, you come to the second major section, which tries to describe the actual practice of medicine, in its many branches. If your bent is not in the main a scientific one, you may find this section (chapters 4–6) more interesting, and you may even wonder why I did not begin with it. The answer is that (in my view at least) too much has been written about the 'human' side of medicine, with little appreciation of the importance of concrete medical knowledge. In chapter 1 I hope to explain how we need both sides, the scientific and the human, in our approach to medicine; they are simply two ways of looking at things, and we need them both, in different circumstances. Just at present, however, there seems to me a greater danger of neglecting the scientific aspect, which is why I am putting it first.

In the third section (chapters 7–9), I discuss those aspects of medicine which deal not with the care of individual patients, but with the health of populations; and still more broadly with the ways in which health services can be provided, and the relationship between medicine and society in general.

At the end of the book, there is a limited glossary, and suggestions for further reading.

This book was commissioned by Miss Kim Pickin, who has kept in touch with it chapter by chapter, with suggestions and encouragement. I have a very particular obligation to my former colleague in Manchester, Dr John Swales, now the Foundation Professor of Medicine in the Leicester Medical School. He kindly agreed to my request that if anything should prevent me from completing the writing of this book, he should take over. I am of course happy that this has so far not proved necessary; but I remain deeply in his debt for his helpful and very pertinent comments on the chapters as they have appeared. He has saved me from a number of egregious errors; any which remain are attributable to me alone. I am also much indebted to the Wellcome Trust, and to their Director, Dr P. O. Williams, for their continued support, and I am particularly grateful for the secretarial work of Mrs Jean Shephard, who has prepared the entire typescript.

PART I

The Nature of Medical Knowledge

1

What is Medicine?

You may recall Mr Punch's advice to those about to marry – 'Don't'. My own advice to those who are about to take up medical study, and who are qualified to do so, would be the exact opposite – 'By all means, do.' Such positive encouragement can only be given by someone who firmly believes in the future of medicine and can only be justified by some understanding of the nature of medicine, and of the exceptional, perhaps even unique, variety of opportunities it offers to men and women of widely differing character and capacity.

We all know in a general way what medicine is about – to preserve health and either to cure illness or at least relieve its consequences. It does not take a five- or six-year university course to teach these objectives; but the means of attaining them demand prolonged and intensive study, refreshed from time to time during a working life to take account of important extensions to the field of what is medically possible. Later chapters will describe in some detail how doctors usually work but in this introductory chapter I shall try to pick out some of the features common to all branches of the medical profession.

MEDICINE AS A PROFESSION

First, what is implied in describing medicine as a *profession*? It implies *recognized standards* of training and qualification and adherence to *ethical obligations* whose essence is to place the interests of the client, in this case the patient, above one's own. These are exacting criteria, certainly not reached at all times, in all places and by all; but nevertheless they are worthy ideals, and progress towards them is encouraged, and if necessary enforced, in Britain by the General Medical Council, and by comparable bodies in many other countries.

The General Medical Council is a statutory body, in large part elected by the profession, but also with members appointed by educational bodies and by government. It has a statutory responsibility for monitoring standards of undergraduate and postgraduate medical training, to which end it approves curricula and inspects courses and examinations. It does not itself conduct examinations, but it maintains a register of those who are medically qualified and this register is publicly available. In those exceptional cases where doctors flagrantly break the civil or criminal law, or commit 'serious professional misconduct', the Council can warn the practitioner, can suspend him from practice, or can erase or 'strike off' his name from the Register, following which it would be an offence for him to purport to be a medical practitioner, until reinstated on appeal. The term 'serious professional misconduct' has recently been substituted for the harsher-sounding 'infamous conduct in a professional respect'; but in making the change the Council 'intended that the phrases should have the same significance'.

In these disciplinary matters the Council has an influence going far beyond what might be inferred from the small number of actual erasures; for its powers are well known, it considers many cases that do not lead to the more extreme sanctions and it issues positive recommendations on fitness to practice. Wisely, in my view, the Council does not set out a formal *code of practice*, though such codes have been attempted since the time of Hippocrates. The Council can only lay down a minimum standard; it cannot in a general statement take account of varied, but still permissible, ethical standpoints both of the doctor and of the patient; moreover any such statement is liable to be outmoded by rapid changes in what is possible in medicine and what is legally

4

permissible, or generally sanctioned, in society. As a concrete example, consider abortion, which was both an offence and a ground for erasure from the Register until 1967, when it was made legal under certain conditions by the Abortion Act 1967. The new law was far from straightforward, however, and did not solve all the practical problems, to some extent replacing one set of problems by another.

We shall come back to the ethical aspects of medicine in later chapters; ethics is mentioned here simply as one of the marks of a profession. A long and arduous training and high standards of professional conduct may at first glance seem to be deterrents to the student contemplating medicine, but they are of great advantage, both to the public and to doctors themselves. Professional status, and the training and standards which it implies, are things to be cherished.

SCIENCE AND ART

The second mark of medicine is that it combines *scientific knowledge* with the *communicative skills* necessary for dealing with patients. We are of course talking of ideals here, admirably summarized in the motto of the Royal College of General Practitioners, 'Cum scientia caritas', which might be loosely and clumsily translated as 'Loving-kindness in the exercise of scientifically based practical skills'. I think it is a great mistake to try to attach priorities to these two different elements of medical practice – they are both important and they must be kept in balance. I would ask those who undervalue the scientific aspect of modern medical practice to think what medicine was like 100 or even 50 years ago. Read accounts of how illnesses were treated until quite recently and ask what has made the difference. Both public health and individual clinical practice have been pervaded by science, both in its questioning aspect and also in the certainties – yes, certainties – which science attains from time to time. When I qualified, of five young patients with pneumonia, one would die; and tuberculosis was still the recognized captain of the men of death. Of course, people still die; but it is now rare for this to happen in childhood or in early adult life, tragic though such happenings individually still are. So I would say to such detractors, think again about what medical practice could be like without its scientific basis.

On the other hand, it is equally possible to be so dazzled by the objective achievements of medical science as to undervalue what may be called the human or humane element in medicine, that towards which Hippocrates was pointing when he said, 'Where there is love of mankind, there is also love of the art'. It is easy for the practising doctor, and perhaps particularly for the academic, to become impatient with those who speak of 'whole person' medicine, or 'holistic' medicine, as if personal relationships did not lie at the heart of all clinical medicine. But to anyone who sees the future of medicine solely in terms of scientific progress, I would point out that both in relation to the public health and in the individual practice of medicine, the most difficult part of the whole enterprise may be to disentangle those aspects to which science can properly be applied from the surrounding matrix of vested interests and individual fears. This calls for subtlety in human relations, which must both precede, and later follow, the strictly scientific part of the analysis. Otherwise, in public health what is scientifically desirable may turn out to be publicly unacceptable; and in individual practice, the patient may openly or covertly fail to accept the advice given to him, however scientifically valid it may be. This phenomenon of 'non-compliance' is not one-sided, and it may be at least as much the fault of the doctor as of the patient.

Although I have outlined two extreme positions here, I do find it quite hard to believe that there are many with actual experience of medical practice who conceive of it either as 'pure art' or as 'pure science'. Even in the general population, and certainly from my experience in the university world, I very much doubt whether there exist on the one hand pure artistic persons who have no liking for practical affairs, or on the other hand pure scientists who have no use for other people, or for art and music. But if such people do exist, they certainly should not be doctors in any practical sense, for it is the coming together of scientific knowledge and human sympathy which is the only proper basis of medical practice.

The synthesis of science and sympathy which I believe to be central to the practice of medicine can be looked at in another way, if we adopt a well-known analysis of what is needed for practice as 'knowledge, skills and attitudes'. 'Knowledge' is the theoretical component of medicine, to which science makes the major contribution, particularly if we include the behavioural sciences. 'Skills' are the practical procedures which doctors are trained to carry out, some of which, like competent history-taking, are needful for all practising doctors; while others, like surgery, may be the province of particular specialties. However, knowledge and skills may both be present in high degree, but may still be corrupted by faulty attitudes, or reinforced by good attitudes. Attitudes are of course partly an individual matter, but they are greatly reinforced, and in extreme cases controlled, by the corporate attitudes accepted by the profession as a whole.

SPECIALIZATION

So far I have been emphasizing those important elements of professional standards and ethics, and the union of scientific knowledge and human sympathy, which are common to all branches of medical practice. The mention of 'specialties' in the paragraph above prompts me now to comment on the wide variety of careers to which a qualification in medicine opens the door. The very broad divisions of medical practice are general or family practice, the largest single branch, the various hospital specialties and the 'community physicians', whose main concern is with the health of populations and the organization of services. Yet within these broad groupings there is great variety. For the general practitioners, there is diversity of environment from the inner city to the remote rural districts; and diversity of organization, from individual practice to a group practice or health centre with computerized records and a team of associates. For the hospital specialist (and for his patients) the variety is bewildering. Surgery, medicine, psychiatry and obstetrics are only the beginning; there are over 20 recognized specialties and associated training programmes within internal medicine, and somewhat similar specialization within surgery (see Appendix). 'Community medicine' is also something of a blanket term, including administrative medicine, environmental medicine, epidemiology, school medical clinics and so on; and there is the increasingly important specialty of occupational medicine, which is, in a particular context, something of a bridge between clinical medicine and public health. There is of course more to be said on these various branches of medicine; but the point to be made for the present is that there is a sufficient range of occupations within medicine to content anyone who is capable of contentment.

In this opening chapter I have taken a rather 'high', idealistic view of medicine because I believe that to be the proper one, and one which is more likely to produce good doctors. It is a view that stresses duties more than rights for the doctor, advice rather than 'orders' for the patient and the objective content of medical work rather than the 'role-playing' ascribed to doctors by some students of society. I do not myself warm to the view of the doctor-patient relationship as one between adversaries, a view sometimes consciously or unconsciously encapsulated in the phrase 'the clinical encounter'. Nor do I readily see the doctor as 'an agent of society', reducing people by means of 'labelling' into an acceptance of 'the sick role'. Certainly, the practice of medicine can be looked on as itself providing a role for the doctor, as a means of social regulation and as a way of making money – not a fortune, but still a substantial amount. Surely it is better to encourage the clinical doctor to give his priority to helping the individual patient and the community physician to be, in Virchow's★ phrase, 'the natural advocate of the poor'; and in each doctor, whatever his particular vocation, there should be some openness to both these objectives.

★ Rudolf Virchow (1821–1902). German pathologist, the father of 'cellular pathology' (see chapter 3). Also a pioneer of social medicine, a member of the Prussian Diet and an anthropologist.

2

Health and Disease

It is interesting to note that the Greeks placed medicine in the care not of one protective deity, but of two – Hygeia and Asclepius – one looking to the preservation of health, the other to the cure of disease. To make a rigid distinction between prevention and cure, however, is to ignore that they have a common basis in medical knowledge, and that as we go through life we all of us are likely to have need of both. It is of little comfort to the victim of a lung tumour to tell him that 20 years ago he should not have begun to smoke, however true such a statement might be; by the time he complains of his chest, his need is for surgery if possible, and if not for medical relief of symptoms and support for himself and his family. The promotion of health and the prevention of disease are two sides of the same coin. We are given at birth, or rather at conception, a potential for healthy development; we then become subject to an array of environmental influences which may make or mar our inherent endowment of health.

The relative contribution of genetic and environmental factors to health and disease is perhaps not as controversial as the relative contribution of these factors to intelligence, which is debated as much from the standpoint of political preconception as from any conclusive scientific evidence. The protagonists fall into two camps: on the whole 'soft-liners' place greater weight on environmental factors, in the hope that these can be more easily modified to the good; while 'hard-liners' place greater emphasis on our genetic stock, and in extreme cases almost seem to deprecate any reduction in evolutionary pressure stemming from improving the environment, fearing that we 'may become soft'. Without subscribing to its total realism, my own leaning is towards the slogan of the World Health Organisation (WHO), 'Health for all by the year 2000', coupled with its definition of health as 'a state of complete physical, mental and social well-being, and not merely the absence of disease or infirmity'. As George Herbert (1593–1633) put it, 'He shoots higher that threatens the moon than he that aims at a tree'.

In spite of this declaration of faith in the possibilities of piecemeal social engineering directed towards improvement in health status, I do not foresee an early resolution of the broad conflict of principle between emphasis on heredity and emphasis on the environment. However, it does not matter too much to the developed plant what contribution it owes to soil and what to the seed; and it is perhaps time to consider more specific matters. In the remainder of this chapter, I shall summarize some of the particular genetic and environmental influences on our health.

GENETIC INFLUENCES ON HEALTH

The proverbial Martian visiting this planet would certainly be impressed by the wide variation in physical characteristics within any group he encountered; and he might also notice that there was less variation between brothers and between sisters than among men and women at large. Putting these two things together, he might conclude that there is a considerable inherited component in such things as our stature, our facial appearance and the colour of our eyes and hair. (The degree to which inherited characteristics are actually expressed in the individual can of course be altered by environmental factors, such as a period of undernutrition during childhood.) Pursuing his inquiries further, he might learn that some physical characteristics, such as brown or blue colour of the iris, have a definite pattern of inheritance, with brown colour being 'dominant'; while other characteristics, such as stature, show no similarly clear-cut pattern and are described as 'polygenic' or 'multifactorial'.

In his monastery at Brno, the Abbé Mendel patiently unravelled the first part of the story of genetic variation, the raw material on which natural selection acts to bring about the evolutionary progress delineated by Wallace and Darwin. The chemical anatomy of genetic material remained to be discovered by Watson and Crick, opening up long vistas of molecular biology, extending as far as genetic manipulation by recombinant DNA technology. This exciting field of science belongs strictly to biology rather than to medicine, but its fruits are already available to medical practice in the production of human-type insulin, of interferon, and of monoclonal antibodies.

The genetic factors that determine such things as our stature and the colour of our eyes do not influence our state of health, so far as present knowledge goes; but there are genetic factors that do, and they do so in various ways. Just as with physical characteristics, some genetically induced illnesses have a clear-cut pattern of inheritance, whereas others are multifactorial.

Some genetically determined conditions arise anew, either from mutation of a gene, or from abnormal chromosome formation, such as the additional chromosome 21 which is the basis of some forms of Down's syndrome (formerly called mongolism). Other conditions pass from generation to generation, following the various patterns of Mendelian inheritance. Thus, they may be *dominant*, and affect both sexes, such as the gene responsible for the type of muscle disease known as dystrophia myotonica. They may be *recessive*, attaining expression only in the absence of a corresponding normal gene, a circumstance which may arise when two carriers marry, and is thus favoured by inbreeding. A very characteristic pattern of inheritance is manifested by the relatively trivial condition of red–green colour blindness, and by the dangerous bleeding disorder, haemophilia, which notoriously affected some of the royal families of

Europe, including the tsarevich Alexis, who was mistreated by Rasputin.

In haemophilia, the abnormal gene lies in the X chromosome, and is recessive. In females, with their XX constitution, the abnormal gene is balanced by the normal gene on the X chromosome derived from the normal father; such a female would still, like her mother, be a carrier of the disease, but would not herself experience it. But her male children would have an equal chance of receiving from her a normal or an abnormal X chromosome; if one of them were unfortunate enough to receive the latter, since his constitution is XY, the abnormal gene would not be matched by a normal gene, and he would suffer from haemophilia.

So long as haemophilia was likely to prove fatal during childhood, the 'simple' pattern of female carriers and male victims persisted; but the availability of blood transfusion and later of anti-haemophilic globulin now allows survival of affected males to reproductive age. If such a man should himself marry a carrier, the daughters of that marriage would have a 50 per cent chance of actually suffering from haemophilia, the other 50 per cent being 'merely' carriers. Real life, however, is not always obedient to theory, and the patterns of Mendelian inheritance may be obscured if the genetic predisposition fails to show itself in actual disease, a phenomenon known as 'incomplete penetrance'.

To recap, I have outlined two major groups of genetic disorders, those due to *gross abnormalities in the chromosomes*, such as Down's syndrome and various deviations from the normal XX (female) or XY (male) constitution which may lead to disparity between genetic or 'true' sex and external appearances; and those due to *single abnormal genes*, sometimes known as 'Mendelian or simply inherited disorders'. The 'simplicity' does not of course imply any deep understanding of what causes these genetic anomalies, nor even a single pattern. Far from it, for this group can be further subdivided into three.

The first group are called '*autosomal dominant disorders*'. They are due to a single abnormal gene on a chromosome other than X or Y. Examples include such conditions as polycystic renal disease, neurofibromatosis and Huntington's chorea. Since these are serious conditions, and since on average half the children of an affected parent will also be affected, the question arises why such conditions do not 'die out'. The likely explanation differs in different conditions. Sometimes, although a family history shows it to be dominant, the condition is incompletely expressed; or, as in the case of polycystic renal disease or Huntington's chorea, clinical expression is delayed until an age before which reproduction may well have occurred. Other dominant disorders, such as neurofibromatosis, are prevented from extinction by a high rate of mutation, that is, new abnormal genes arise to replace those lost by the death of affected patients.

The second group are the '*autosomal recessive disorders*', due to the conjunction of two abnormal autosomal genes, one derived from each parent. Since the carrier state ordinarily confers no disadvantage to the health of the carrier, it may be relatively common, as with sickle-cell anaemia in certain populations. Another relatively common autosomal dominant disorder is cystic fibrosis; but other such conditions, e.g. albinism and phenylketonuria, are rare.

'*X-linked disorders*', the third group, are due to an abnormal gene on the X chromosome, which gives the characteristic pattern of inheritance described above for haemophilia. Other conditions with this form of inheritance are a rare form of rickets associated with low phosphate levels in the blood and deficiency of an enzyme (glucose 6-phosphate dehydrogenase) which makes affected people react abnormally to some drugs by breaking down some of their red blood cells.

The great majority of these conditions with clear-cut inheritance are rare, but they are of course of great importance to the affected families and individuals. More-over, there are well over a thousand such conditions, so taken all together the number of people involved is considerable. Nevertheless, the main burden of genetically related disease arises not from these clear-cut disorders, but from much commoner conditions which 'run in families', such as essential hypertension (raised blood pressure), diabetes mellitus arising in later life and schizophrenia. These important *multifactorial genetic diseases* show a concentration of cases within families, but there is no clear-cut Mendelian pattern of inheritance such as would suggest that only one or at most two abnormal genes were sufficient to cause the condition. The concept of multiple, presumably minor, gene abnormalities is conveyed in the term 'polygenic inheritance', and analogy can be drawn with the inheritance of physical characteristics, and probably of intelligence. In the clear-cut genetic disorders, the paramount importance of genetic factors is obvious; but in the polygenic disorders, it becomes much more difficult to assess the balance between genetic and environmental factors. For example, essential hypertension has been variously regarded as a graded characteristic, like stature, for example, inherited polygenically; as a disease related to a dominant gene but with a low rate of expression (perhaps something of a contradiction in terms); and as the result of stress, a term not too rigorously defined. The first two of these views were vigorously argued for more than a decade by George Pickering and Robert Platt. After the noise of battle, it now seems likely that in scientific terms Pickering was right in regarding essential hypertension as a graded characteristic, with polygenic inheritance; but pragmatically the two antagonists would unite in treating the upper levels of blood pressure with hypotensive drugs. The problem of a cut-off point above which treatment should be given, and below which it need not be, remains with us; since treatment is for life, in more than one sense, the decision is not a light one.

The importance of a genetic component in a number of diseases has received interesting support from developments in tissue-typing, whose original purpose was to diminish the likelihood of rejection of organs such as kidneys transplanted from one individual to another. Such rejection is due to the immune system of the recipient recognizing certain components of the donor's tissue as 'foreign' and mounting a reaction to them; these components are known as the 'histocompatibility antigens', and they belong to a complex system known as the HLA system. These antigens are genetically determined by genes in a specific region of chromosome 6, and they can be characterized by their reaction with specific antisera. Characteristic HLA profiles have now been demonstrated in a number of diseases of joints, skin and endocrine glands not previously known to have a genetic component. The strength of the association varies from one disease to another, but its existence does validate the genetic component, while its inconstancy demonstrates the importance of environmental factors in modifying what is inherited.

I hope that, however baldly, I may have indicated that studies of the mechanism of inheritance by biochemical and immunological methods constitute one of the most exciting and rapidly developing fields of biology; and also that these studies have relevance to human (and also to animal) disease, a relevance reflected in the medical discipline of clinical genetics. Doctors and scientists specializing in this field work on the elucidation and care of a host of heritable disorders, and provide counselling services for would-be parents with a family history of genetic disorder. A similarly close relationship between basic science and clinical practice could be illustrated in many other areas, and is indeed a hallmark of good modern medicine.

Of course, the problems posed by the large group of heritable disorders cannot be solved by science alone. For the clear-cut answers which science may appear to give have to be matched with the ethical standards of society and those of the prospective parents. The doctor's place, in my view, is to describe the possible choices to the parents as clearly as he can; to discuss the situation but not to impose his own ethical preconceptions at the expense of theirs. Any action taken must, of course, come within the law of the land, and within recognized codes of ethical practice; but even these are subject to change. Termination of pregnancy which was both illegal and condemned by medical codes of ethics since Hippocrates, was made legal under certain safeguards not too long ago, and medical disciplinary procedures had to conform to the new legal position. In these difficult issues,

16

codes of practice may be helpful as guidelines, but some latitude must still remain to take account of the infinite variety of considerations relevant to any particular cases.

ENVIRONMENTAL INFLUENCES ON HEALTH

Some of these are so inescapably obvious as to be matters of common knowledge. If we are deprived of oxygen for more than a few minutes we suffer irreversible brain damage, and shortly die. If we are deprived of water and other beverages, we die in a few days, earlier in hot climes; and if deprived of food, but not of water, we may live for a month or two, but no longer. There are, however, more subtle influences of environment on health, and some of these were already known to the Greeks. The Hippocratic writings contain an essay on 'Airs, Waters, Places', with a characteristic combination of sound sense and unverified supposition. For example:

The best water comes from high ground and hills covered with earth. This is sweet and clear and, when taken with wine, but little wine is needed to make a palatable drink. Moreover, it is cool in summer and warm in winter because it comes from very deep springs. I particularly recommend water which flows towards the east, and even more that which flows towards the north-east, since it is very sparkling, sweet-smelling and light. Water that is salty, hard and cannot be softened, is not always good to drink.

On the other hand, 'A man who is in good and robust health need not distinguish between them [waters], but he may drink whatever is to hand at the moment.'

When we come to the scientific study of environmental influences on health, we find interesting resemblances and differences between that study and the study of genetic influences. To take the resemblance first, in both of them there is essential continuity between basic science and practical application. In the case of genetic factors, I have already stressed the link between basic genetics, itself

17

supported by biochemistry and immunology, and clinical genetics, which of course contributes to basic knowledge in addition to benefiting from it. For environmental factors, the analogous disciplines are statistics on the one hand and clinical epidemiology on the other. Basic statistical theory has benefited greatly from the work of such as Pascal, Galton and Karl Pearson, who also had a strong interest in practical applications; conversely, clinical epidemiology depends on making simple but informed observation subject to the rigours of statistics.

There is, however, quite an important difference between our knowledge of genetic and of environmental factors in health and disease. The sciences basic to clinical genetics and to clinical epidemiology could both, it is true, fall within the usual understanding of 'an exact science', but when it comes to application, for chromosome anomalies and for Mendelian inheritance at least, there is enough established fact to allow the making of categorical statements, some of which I have already made in the first part of this chapter. When we pass from individuals to populations (and that is what we are doing in passing from clinical medicine to clinical epidemiology) the subject matter of our study changes, and loses definition; consequently the statements we can make about it tend to be based on probabilities rather than categorical. This does not, of course, imply any sort of hierarchy in the applied sciences – on the one hand, a probabilistic statement may still be a very strong one, with probability approaching unity; while on the other hand, a categorical statement may turn out to be in error, as further knowledge accrues. Moreover, in practical terms, it is just as important to know that there is a very high probability that people who drink heavily increase their chance of getting liver disease, though without any certainty of their doing so, as it is to know that a dominant trait will affect half the children of a marriage (and of course we do not know which half). What we have here is a virtual certainty for the 'group', but only a probability for the 'individual'.

Prenatal influences

Although the uterine environment is something of a special case, the period of some nine months between conception and birth is a critical period. Some of the relatively high incidence of spontaneous abortion (miscarriage) – just under 15 per cent – is accounted for by major chromosome abnormalities and by lethal mutation; but this is far from being the whole story, since women suffering from recurrent spontaneous abortion are as a rule carrying normal fetuses. Evidence is accruing that the likelihood of spontaneous abortion in this syndrome can be reduced by injecting lymphocytes taken from the father, and this would indicate that the cause of the trouble was in the uterine environment rather than in the fetus itself.

Other clear-cut influences of the uterine environment on the fetus are the occurrence of deafness, eye troubles and heart malformations in some of the offspring of mothers who had rubella (German measles) in early pregnancy; and the severe damage to the red blood cells of Rhesus-positive infants born to Rhesus-negative mothers who have developed antibodies to Rhesus-positive cells. This very serious type of haemolytic anaemia is now preventable, thanks to the work of Cyril Clarke and his colleagues in Liverpool. The problem arises because at the time of birth, small amounts of fetal blood containing Rh-positive cells may pass into the mother's circulation; if she is Rh-negative, she may develop antibodies to the Rhesus factor, which could then damage a subsequent Rh-positive fetus. This sequence can, however, be prevented by injecting the mother with potent antibody to Rh-positive cells at the time of delivery. This will destroy any contaminating Rh-positive cells before they have had time to stimulate the mother to become sensitized to Rh-positive cells.

In addition to these relatively clear-cut conditions, many congenital physical abnormalities and also mental subnormality may be due to prenatal influences, and also of course to accidents at birth. As McKeown puts it, 'These diseases are attributable to unknown influences within the uterus operating on genetic material whose character is also obscure'. As McKeown has also pointed out, the generality of congenital disorders are thus determined prenatally and are not susceptible to prevention; but there are possibilities of the kind mentioned above, together with the more radical preventive measures of genetic counselling and selective induced abortion of fetuses established as having serious anomalies which would threaten both the duration and quality of their lives. For example, by a combination of chemical screening, ultrasound examination and amniocentesis it is possible to detect anencephaly and spina bifida early in pregnancy; the parents can then be advised of the situation, but the ultimate decision must rest with them. Indeed, it is wise before setting out on a trail of investigation to make sure that at the end of the road the parents will consider the possibility of termination; this is not an issue which should be forced on parents.

The general environment

Pure air, good food and clean water stand out as the simple necessities of life; but as with freedom, their price in developed countries is eternal vigilance and in the developing countries good food and clean water may be sadly lacking, basic though they are to good health.

Pure air, like sunlight, comes free in nature; but in an industrial society there is the risk of contamination by smoke, by airborne radioactive particles, by the acid products of combustion of fossil fuels and by a host of chemical pollutants generated in industry. This is a very difficult area in which to maintain perspective, and it may be that some single-issue pressure groups, such as that on lead in petrol, may have over-interpreted the evidence. On the other hand, it is important that control measures for pollutants with known harmful biological effects, such as radioactive materials, should be stringently enforced, and reviewed from time to time. For the readers of Dickens, and especially for anyone old enough to remember the 'pea-soupers' of the 1930s and 1940s, the smoke-free zones established following the Clean Air Acts are an indication that we are capable of improving our environment in the sphere of atmospheric pollution.

Clean water is again something that we take for granted. The last big epidemic of cholera in Britain was in 1865. The other major water-borne disease, typhoid or enteric fever, remained a serious health problem until the turn of the century, although it only reached major proportions during military operations. In many parts of the world, however, cholera and typhoid remain major sources of morbidity and mortality. In striving to eliminate them, the World Health Organisation rightly lays emphasis on the provision of a clean water supply, which is both more acceptable and more effective than immunization against these particular diseases.

The provision of good food requires attention to quantity – neither too little nor too much – but also to much more. Raw materials of good quality must be stored in such a way as to prevent the growth of fungi, with their aflatoxins which are an important cause of liver damage in the tropics; they must be handled cleanly, to prevent contamination with bacteria, or with their toxins, some of which are not destroyed by heat. There must be a balance among protein, carbohydrate and fat; and there must be adequate but not excessive amounts of minerals and vitamins. Nutritional evidence is not always conclusive, however fervently propagated; but there is a likelihood that in the recent past in developed countries we have been eating too much fat, too much meat, too much sugar, too much salt and not enough cereal, fruit and vegetables in their natural state – the fibre-containing foods. But there is an element of conjecture in these matters, and one has to be cautious in giving advice both to populations and to individuals. One complication is that some 'good' foods, like fruit and vegetables, are expensive; but fortunately others, such as bread, are relatively cheap. When it comes to individuals, the fairly high prevalence of individual intolerances to specific foods, or to food additives, has to be kept in mind. Not only primary producers, but also food processors and food distributors have a responsibility for providing nutritionally good food, and for labelling it so that people can at least know what they are eating. With the general interest in food, there has been some improvement in this direction, with an increase in the range of foods now available in food stores.

Life-style and health

I believe the benefits of civilization, including those bestowed on us by applied science, far outweigh its drawbacks, even including what are sometimes termed 'the diseases of civilization'. This term is commonly used to denote conditions such as 'heart attacks', which are not confined to civilized societies, but are believed to be more prevalent within them. This may be partly a matter of ascertainment, for example it was long believed that sprue* affected only expatriate Europeans in India, until one day someone started looking for it in Indians! It may also be that, with diseases that occur mainly in later life, an increased prevalence in civilized societies is related to the greater number of people remaining alive long enough to experience them. I for one would not readily exchange our present 'civilized' conditions for those of a 'state of nature', so succinctly described by Thomas Hobbes: 'No art; no letters; no society; and which is worst of all, continual fear and danger of violent death; and the life of man, solitary, poor, nasty, brutish and short.' If survival be a measure of health (and they must somehow be correlated), then over the past century or more we have undoubtedly been faring better, and not worse. In 1841, the male death rate per 1,000 was about 23 and the female about 21; in 1971 the corresponding figures were 8 and 5, respectively and approximately.

No doubt many factors have contributed to this general increase in survival. They are likely to include an improved standard of nutrition, reflected among other things in an increase in stature; better housing, which in conjunction

* A form of fatty diarrhoea (or steatorrhoea) found mainly in the tropics.

with the more recent tendency to smaller families, has diminished the spread of infection; clean water supply and effective sewage disposal, which greatly diminished fatal intestinal infections. More recently, there have been advances both in preventive and in curative medicine which must have made some contribution, though opinions differ as to the importance of this at the population level. Personally, and perhaps naturally, I would regard it as important, even at that level; and at the individual level, in specific diseases, there can be little doubt of its importance.

Of course, the fact that on average we are living longer in no way rules out that there may still be adverse factors in our life-style. There is hard medical evidence that the use of tobacco to any extent, and the use of alcohol in excess (a quantity which the individual tends to judge for himself) confer serious disadvantages to health and survival. Failure to take a reasonable amount of exercise also contributes to obesity and probably to 'heart attacks'. The influence of 'the stress of modern life' I find difficult to assess. Primitive societies living under the threat of starvation, and perhaps fleeing from beasts of prey, must have offered elements of stress. However, Wilfred Trotter and others have pointed out the distinction between spontaneous behaviour in response to clear-cut personal stimuli and the more complex behaviour in response to social norms, which is less 'natural', and may thus give rise to greater stress. Personally, I remain to be convinced that primitive 'fight or flight' was any less of a health hazard than 'nail-biting worry', except in so far as the latter tends to be sedentary.

Psychological and social factors

So far, we have been considering relatively tangible genetic and environmental influences on health. It is more difficult to assess the influence of psychological factors. These cannot be measured directly, as is the case with some physical factors although progress has been made with the various tests of intelligence, and with assessments of psychological disturbance by such means as the General Health

Questionary, devised by David Goldberg, and now widely used. However, much psychodynamic activity never comes to the surface and thus cannot be directly assessed, but that in no way excludes it from being a potent cause of disease and suffering. Whatever the relationship between the psyche (mind) and the soma (body), and indeed whether they are separate as Descartes supposed (i.e. mind–body dualism), or indissolubly linked as common sense might suggest, there can be little doubt that they function interdependentally. Adverse life situations such as bereavement and mental distress in general are reflected in physical manifestations, which may by their intensity and duration qualify for the label of 'disease'. Equally, the strains of life may precipitate the overt onset of mental disorders such as schizophrenia. Conversely, physical illness, especially if it be both painful and prolonged, as may happen with neuralgia following shingles in the elderly, can lead to profound depression. The term 'psychosomatic illness' is sometimes applied to conditions such as ulcerative colitis or peptic ulcer, where the balance between psychological and physical factors may be apparent over a long period; but I am not sure of the validity of separating off one group of disorders from within a spectrum which ranges from the predominantly physical, such as accident or acute illness, to the predominantly psychological, such as depression appearing out of an apparently cloudless sky. Another argument, should one be necessary, for the closeness of interaction between the physical and the psychological arises from the effects of drugs, including alcohol, on mood and behaviour. On the other hand, a good doctor does not forget to include comfort in his armamentarium for 'organic' disease, difficult though it may at times be to administer.

The importance of the crises of life in precipitating both mental and physical illnesses has just been mentioned. Such catastrophes may fall most heavily on those least able to bear them, and this may be one of the factors determining the high morbidity and mortality among unskilled manual workers, compared with the professional classes. At these extremes, the difference is considerable, the relative mortality in 'social class V' being between two and four times that in 'social class I' at different ages, the discrepancy being greatest in the first year after birth. The health experience of the classes lying between I and V shows the expected gradient, perhaps particularly clearly in another index of health status, maternal mortality.

A few years ago, I and some able colleagues had the opportunity to study this phenomenon in some depth; the results were published.* Our main conclusion was that the poor health of the 'lower social classes' was the result of economic deprivation, which brings a constellation of disadvantages relevant to health, which include poor nutrition, poor housing, lack of safe play areas for children and overcrowding which favours the spread of infection. Our assumption that social deprivation leads to ill-health can of course be challenged, and even turned on its head, by taking the view that ill-health leads to social deprivation. While that is no doubt true in specific cases, the amount of mobility known to occur upwards or downwards between the social classes is insufficient to support the idea of a 'downward movement of the unfit' as being the sole, or even a major, cause of health inequality. While recognizing that they were of importance in specific cases, we also did not accept either the health hazards of specific occupations, or difficulties in access to medical care, as major factors in explaining the relatively poor health of social classes IV and V. We did, however, draw attention to the poor uptake of preventive measures by those in social classes IV and V, and to the higher prevalence of smoking among them. We had to admit that complete abolition of this type of inequality in health would require the abolition of poverty, which might be an expensive business, but at least a start should be made in improving the lot of pregnant mothers and their children, as an investment for the future. I quote here the central paragraph of our summary, as a supplement to the gloss I have already given.

* Townsend, P. & Davidson, N., *Inequalities in Health*, Penguin, Harmondsworth, 1982.

We do not believe there to be any single and *simple explanation* of the complex data we have assembled. While there are a number of quite distinct theoretical approaches to explanation we wish to stress the importance of differences in material conditions of life. *In our view much of the evidence on social inequalities in health can be adequately understood in terms of specific features of the socio-economic environment*: features (such as work accidents, overcrowding, cigarette smoking) which are strongly class-related in Britain and also have clear causal significance. Other aspects of the evidence indicate the importance of the health services and particularly preventive services. Ante-natal care is probably important in preventing perinatal death, and the international evidence suggests that much can be done to improve ante-natal care and its uptake. But beyond this there is undoubtedly much which cannot be understood in terms of the impact of so specific factors, but only in terms of the more diffuse consequences of the class structure: poverty, working conditions, and deprivation in its various forms. It is this acknowledgement of the *multicausal* nature of health inequalities, within which inequalities in the material conditions of living loom large, which informs and structures our policy recommendations. These draw also upon another aspect of our interpretation of the evidence. We have concluded that early childhood is the period of life at which intervention could most hopefully weaken the continuing association between health and class. There is, for example, abundant evidence that inadequately treated bouts of childhood illness 'cast long shadows forward', as the Court Committee put it.

This general account of the genetic and environmental influences on health has necessarily been illustrated by the mention of a number of specific diseases, but there has been no general account of 'disease' as such. In the next chapter I will examine the deceptively simple question of what is a disease, and look at some examples of disease processes.

3

What is Disease?

There are two views of disease which are, at least superficially, contrasting. One view is that it does not really exist, and this conforms to what has been called 'the social model'. The other view is that it does, and this is referred to, with occasionally a suspicion of distaste, as 'the medical model'. A paper prepared some years ago for what was then the Social Science Research Council, and has now (a sign of the times?) become the Economic and Social Research Council characterizes these two models more fully, in the form of a table of contrasting characteristics:

Medical model	Social model
Individual	Population
Treatment	Prevention
Cure	Care
Medical	Social
Hospital	Community
Acute	Chronic

With respect (as civil servants say when they are about to express strong disagreement), I think this is a superficial and misleading analysis, for reasons which I have gone into at greater length in a published lecture which I entitled 'An anthology of false antitheses'.* For now it is enough to say that I believe both models contain elements of the truth, and

* Black, D., *An Anthology of False Antitheses*, Nuffield Provincial Hospitals Trust, London, 1984.

neither of them represents the whole truth. But as a doctor with some experience of practice, it is not surprising if I should lean towards the medical model, and on the whole rebut suggestions that modern medicine is a misdirected activity; that doctors are 'agents of society' condemning patients to 'a sick role' by 'labelling' them; and that the proper business of a health service is to promote health, rather than to concern itself with disease.

I shall return to some of these points later, in considering what is sometimes described, in a grocer-like phrase, as 'the delivery of health care'; but for the present purpose, I have to make a somewhat damaging admission – that diseases do not in fact exist as substantial independent entities. A philosopher would, I think describe this as a 'nominalist' view of disease, in contrast to a 'realist' view; but it would be plainer to say that 'there are no diseases as such, only sick people'. But let me at once go on to say, parodying what Voltaire says of God, that though diseases do not exist as such, it is still necessary to invent them. This is partly for convenience – it improves communication between doctor and patient, and also between doctors and even between patients; for example, it is simpler to say that someone has got pneumonia than to describe the conglomeration of symptoms and signs which have led one to that conclusion. More important, the pragmatic concept of 'disease' is one of the cornerstones of the whole structure of medical knowledge. While it is true that the impact of a harmful agent is different in every individual, this does not destroy the practical utility of identifying the harmful agent, and if possible combating it. To use the concept of 'disease' for purposes of discussion and study does not and should not make us forget the sacred individuality of sick people.

Having as it were (and as I hope) cleared the philosophical ground, let me go on to describe some of the features of disease processes, whose study constitutes the important discipline of 'pathology'.

PATHOLOGY

In the course of a formal training for medical practice, the study of disease processes is preceded by study over a period of two years or more of the normal structure and function of the human body. During these 'preclinical years', as they are called, medical students may become impatient at the mass of detail to which they are exposed, both in anatomy (the structural aspect) and in physiology and biochemistry (the functional aspect). Particularly towards the end of that time, their anxiety, apart of course from passing the examinations in these subjects, is to begin working with real patients. For a thorough understanding of disease processes, however, this solid grounding in normal structure and function is necessary, for we cannot fully understand how things go wrong if we do not know how they work normally in health.

My purpose here is not to give a formal training in pathology, but simply to give some examples of the nature of disease. My concern is thus with what is called 'general pathology' and not with the study of the host of problems that can injure a particular system of the body. Such a study would have to be preceded by a mass of information on the separate characteristics of the various bodily systems which serve the vital purposes of circulation, respiration, digestion, locomotion and so on, together with the nervous sytem and the array of endocrine glands which bind them all together by electrical impulses and by chemical messengers (hormones). That the body has some of the characteristics of a machine creates an opportunity for fruitful study at a certain level, and the products of such study have been momentous; but of course the body is much more than a machine, and the limitations of a reductionist approach (i.e. reducing living processes to chemical or physical terms) have always to be kept in mind. It is a popular fallacy that the care of patients can be likened to the maintenance of a machine, or the replacement of its parts – 'spare-part surgery' is as profoundly misleading an analogy as is 'test tube babies',

29

applied to the culmination of a long process of biological research in which test tubes play no part at all.

LEVELS OF BIOLOGICAL ORGANIZATION

To make it easier to understand the pattern of disease processes I shall introduce at this stage the concept of different levels of biological organization. At the first, *physico-chemical level* the basis of life is a great range of chemical compounds which have in common that among their elementary constituents is carbon. This is a 'tetravalent' element, which means that each atom of carbon can combine with four monovalent atoms, or two divalent atoms. The relatively high valency of the carbon atom opens the door to the tremendous diversity of carbon compounds, of which there are many thousands. It would be possible for life to be based on a tetravalent element other than carbon, such as silicon. For all we know, there may be silicon-based life in other planets – a society of silicon chips, to be fanciful – but what we actually have, at this level, is carbon-based constituents of living matter. We are not, of course, lumps of coal, still less diamonds; and in organic compounds carbon is combined with other elements, most commonly hydrogen, oxygen and nitrogen, but also with sulphur and phosphorus.

There are three major classes of organic compounds which together form the bulk of tissue, apart from water and mineral compounds. These are carbohydrates (the sugars and starches), fats (both saturated and unsaturated), both of which classes contain hydrogen and oxygen together with carbon, and the third class, proteins, which contain nitrogen as well. In addition to proteins, which are made up of chains of amino acids, there is another very important class of nitrogen-containing compounds, the nucleic acids, which include deoxyribonucleic acid (DNA) and ribonucleic acid (RNA). These compounds have importance far out of proportion to their actual amount, for our genetic information is stored in a double helix of DNA: and the translation

30

of genetic information into the constituent proteins of the body is mediated by messenger RNA. This is the situation in higher forms of animal life, while in some bacteria RNA is the bearer of the genetic code.

A tremendous variety of chemical reactions is going on the whole time, ranging from the oxidation of carbohydrates and fats as energy-producing fuels, to the elaboration of complex structural proteins. The detailed study of such reactions is a science in itself, that of *biochemistry*. For our present purpose, it may be enough to say that the speed of these reactions is greatly increased by the presence of catalysts known as enzymes, which are ubiquitous in the tissues of the body; and that some of the important biochemical reactions are both enzyme-dependent and also cyclical, as was first clearly demonstrated by Hans Krebs (1900–81), both for the formation of urea (the ornithine cycle) and for the oxidative production of energy (the tricarboxylic or Krebs cycle). Since each step in such a cycle is enzyme-dependent, the whole cycle is vulnerable to a single enzyme defect. Many enzymes are formed only if the appropriate gene is present; this is one mechanism whereby a genetic defect can produce a specific enzyme defect and this in turn a disorder of metabolism. Although they are mostly very rare, some hundreds of these 'inborn errors of metabolism' are now known, and they form an important group of disorders.

The picture so far may have suggested a welter of biochemical activity, occurring anyhow and anywhere within the body. This is, of course, far from the truth. Not only are some chemical processes specific to particular organs, but there is more generally a structuring of activity within each of the myriad cells of which the body is composed. Many of these are highly specialized to carry out a particular function, but they do have certain structural features in common, constituting the next level of biological organization, that of *subcellular structures*, sometimes known as organelles. The most obvious structural division of a typical cell is between a nucleus, lying more or less in the centre, and the clear cytoplasm which surrounds it. The

nucleus contains the genetic material, organized in chromosomes and genes. The nucleus is affected in, for example,
pernicious anaemia, and also by various drugs used in the
treatment of cancer which affect the metabolism of nucleic
acids. Although it looks clear, the cytoplasm has been
shown by electron microscopy and by other means to have a
complex structure, which to some extent represents biochemical specialization.

Elongated structures known as mitochondria are the main
site of energy production, and they are susceptible to
damage from lack of oxygen. Another intracellular structure
is a network known as the endoplasmic reticulum, which is
particularly concerned with the translation of genetic
information into protein by messenger RNA. Another type
of organelle is the lysosome; these are packets of digestive or
catabolic enzymes which can break down organic compounds. The presence of destructive enzymes may seem
surprising, but within each cell there is a continuous process
of building up and breaking down of material in a dynamic
equilibrium. Damage to the organelles can break down this
equilibrium in various ways.

A region of particular importance to the cell is the
membrane which surrounds it. The fluid within cells differs
quite markedly in composition from the fluid or tissue
matrix which surrounds them; for example, cellular fluid
contains about 20 times as much potassium as does
extracellular fluid, but the situation with sodium is practically the reverse, i.e. much more sodium outside the cells
than inside. These quite striking differences in concentration
are maintained partly by restriction of passage through the
membrane, and partly by energy-dependent pumps which
actively transport sodium and potassium in a direction
contrary to that in which they would naturally travel. When
cells are seriously damaged, or when the membrane is
selectively poisoned, potassium leaks out of the cell, and
sodium seeps in, accompanied by water, so that the cells
become swollen.

As we ascend the ladder of biological organization, the
next landmark we reach is that of the entire cell. Long before

we knew as much as we do now about biochemical processes and fine structure within the cell, the great German pathologist Rudolf Virchow (1821–1902) emphasized the importance of the *cellular level* of organization, in his concept of cellular pathology. Collectively, cells form the bulk of our bodies – some 80 per cent – the remainder being the fluids of the body (blood-plasma★ and the 'tissue fluid' which permeates and moistens our tissues) and to a lesser extent the solid, non-cellular structures in bone and cartilage. The cells in the different tissues of the body can differ greatly in appearance and function. For example, we have the long contractile cells of our muscles; the flattened cells which line the internal passages of our body, and which commonly secrete mucus to protect them from irritants; the cells which secrete digestive enzymes into our gut, and those which secrete regulatory hormones into our bloodstream; and the cells of the nervous sytem which can carry electrical impulses for long distances within the body through extensions of the cells known as axons. But amid all this variety there is a measure of uniformity, in that all cells are vulnerable to such events as cutting off their blood supply, depriving them of oxygen, damaging them physically, exposing them to bacteria, viruses and toxins, and interfering with their function by poisons. While all cells are vulnerable to such processes, both the function and the structural expression of the damage will be modified by the particular properties of the affected cell.

Missing out those local agglomerations of cells known as tissues, which may however be affected by local structural damage from accident or wounding, the next generally significant level of organization is reached with the *physiological system.*

It is not my intention to pre-empt, still less to duplicate, the task of a textbook of medicine by detailing the many ailments which may affect these systems. It is convenient to use a general term, 'lesion', for the harmful effect on

★ Blood-plasma is the liquid component of blood, just over 50 per cent by volume, in which the cells, red and white, are suspended.

structure or on function of a pathological process; thus, the term lesion could embrace a gangrenous toe, which is clearly structural, or the failure of an enzyme, which has functional effects, but still constitutes a biochemical lesion. Lesions of physiological systems can produce both general effects in the body, by impairing a vital function, and also more limited effects, specific to the particular system involved.

I shall give a general indication of the nature and function of the major physiological systems, partly to indicate in concrete terms what is meant by such a system. I shall also mention briefly lesions which are common and which particularly and perhaps interestingly affect a specific system. In no way, however, am I going to attempt an exhaustive treatment of the whole wide field of special pathology.

Circulatory system

Let us give pride of place to this particular system, centred on the heart which from its two ventricles, left and right, drives blood round the body as a whole in the greater circulation and through the lungs in the lesser circulation. Blood leaves the heart in elastic arteries, permeates the various tissues in thin-walled capillaries and returns through veins which have a system of valves to prevent the return to the tissues of blood that has already flowed through them. The blood in the greater circulation carries oxygen and nutrients to the tissues of the body, and removes from them carbon dioxide and waste products. In the lesser circulation to the lungs, the blood is recharged with oxygen and relieved of carbon dioxide.

I find it less surprising that this system sometimes goes wrong than that it normally goes on working for decades, while we remain for the most part unconscious of the heart's effort, repeated every second or oftener. But of course it can go wrong: the possibilities including deformities of the heart or of its valves; interference with the blood supply to the heart itself by narrowing of its own coronary arteries; increased resistance to blood flow because of narrowing of the arteries generally; or, of course, loss of blood from the system by haemorrhage. In addition to general circulatory disturbance, there can also be local blockage of vessels which may lead to cold fingers and toes, or even to gangrene. Sometimes also the clotting of the blood, which is useful in stopping bleeding after a wound, occurs without any good reason, and this can lead to blockage of the veins, with swelling of the feet.

Respiratory system

The circulation and the lungs are partners in ensuring that the tissues are supplied with the oxygen they need for creating energy by the slow combustion of organic material; and for removing the carbon dioxide which is generated in the same process, sometimes described not too happily as 'tissue respiration', where a better term might be 'tissue oxygenation' or 'tissue energy production'. The major process of gas exchange obviously goes on in the lungs, in which millions of tiny air sacs, known as alveoli, are ventilated and then partially emptied during inspiration and expiration. Each alveolus is surrounded by a network of capillaries, which allows rapid diffusion of carbon dioxide from blood to the air in the alveoli, and of oxygen in the opposite direction.

Repeated coughing, either from infective bronchitis or much more commonly from smoking, may over-inflate the alveoli and even rupture their walls, thus impairing the effectiveness of the lungs in the diffusion of gases, which is their prime function. Chronic irritation can also lead to excessive mucus formation. Less commonly, the walls of the alveoli become thickened in disease, again impairing diffusion.

Alimentary system

I prefer this term to the more usual 'digestive system' because digestion is only one element in the process of dealing with food. Food has to be chewed, preferably with a good set of teeth; it is then consciously swallowed, after which the necessary process of propulsion along the course of the gut is unconscious, until the residue arrives at the other end. As we take it in, the food is complex, both physically and chemically; it has to be broken down into small particles and molecules which can be absorbed in the small bowel; the main agents in this are gastric acidity, and the enzymes of stomach, bowel and pancreas, and it is this activity which constitutes digestion proper. Proteins are broken down to their constituent amino-acids, complex starches to simple sugars and fats to fine globules or to their constituent fatty acids and glycerol. Absorption of the different products of digestion then takes place at different levels of the small bowel. Although most nutrients have been absorbed, the material which passes from the small into the large bowel is very fluid; and the main activity of the large bowel is to solidify it by absorbing water and salts.

The alimentary system can be infected, causing vomiting and diarrhoea, which in extreme cases such as cholera can lead to fatal depletion of body fluid within a few hours. More generally, it has great nuisance value in adults, but in infants it is a medical emergency, now fortunately treatable in many cases by giving dilute saline together with some glucose which assists absorption of the saline – a process of oral rehydration which is more practical in tropical countries than the equally effective injected saline. The alimentary tract is a fairly common site of tumours which may cause blockage, leading to vomiting until the obstruction is relieved. A number of conditions can impair absorption, the commonest being a sensitivity reaction to the protein gluten, contained in wheat and other cereals.

Three offshoots of the alimentary tract should be mentioned, though they are functionally distinct from it. The appendix has no known function, but can cause trouble that may necessitate its surgical removal, a life-saving procedure if it has become inflamed or even gangrenous. The pancreas has dual importance; it contributes trypsin and other enzymes to the digestive process, but is also the site of origin of the hormone insulin, vital to the metabolism of glucose.

The liver makes use of the alimentary tract for the drainage of bile, and the bile salts contained therein have a marginal influence on absorption by emulsifying fat particles. The chief function of the liver, however, is metabolic, and it is no exaggeration to call it the major chemical and metabolic factory of the body, both because of its sheer size and because of the complexity of its enzyme systems. Metabolism is something which goes on in all tissues, but it reaches its greatest specialization in the liver. The blood coming from the small bowel, which contains the absorbed products of digestion, passes through the liver before reaching the general circulation, which on the one hand gives the liver the opportunity of modifying what is absorbed, but on the other hand makes it directly accessible to toxic agents, of which alcohol is the most common, and possibly the most important. The liver is also concerned with the modification of many drugs which are given to patients; it may diminish their activity by combining them with other chemical radicals, a process known as conjugation. The enzyme activity in the liver may be enhanced by long term exposure to drugs or alcohol, and this may then diminish the effectiveness of a later drug, because of 'enzyme induction'.

Excretory system

For part of its metabolic activity, the liver can be regarded as part of the excretory system, for it commonly converts both drugs and toxic products of metabolism into inactive derivatives. But the organs most clearly dedicated to excretion are the kidneys, which produce urine, which is then voided via ureters, bladder and urethra. The kidneys are certainly ingenious organs. They are given plenty to work on, for they receive about a fifth of the entire output of the heart, a litre of blood or more each minute. Just over half of this is plasma (the non-cellular part of the blood), and of this they filter about a fifth, giving them each minute about 120 ml of protein-free filtrate, distributed over 2 million separate little filters known as glomeruli. The filtrate makes its way down a tubule, and by far the greater part of it is absorbed on the way down, leaving anywhere from 0.2 to 20 ml of final urine per minute. This apparently cumbrous arrangement is in fact basic to the success of the kidney's operation, for it allows it to respond very selectively to the needs of the body. When we are short of water, the kidney reabsorbs almost all of the original filtrate; while after a large intake of fluid, it can let 100 times as much fluid escape. And it can exercise similar plasticity of function with other constituents. Waste products such as urea are eliminated in concentrated form; whereas other substances may be totally reabsorbed. The regulatory function of the kidney goes hand in hand with its excretory function, and the volume, salt content and acidity of the body fluids are normally kept within rather narrow limits. In a splendid Gallic phrase, Claude Bernard pointed out that it is the constancy of our internal environment which gives freedom to our lives* (in the sense of enabling us to withstand many contrasting environments of temperature, humidity and the like).

The kidneys can be damaged by nephritis or by urinary infection, and in many other ways. Should the damage lead to renal failure, the importance of the regulatory and excretory function which has been lost may be dramatically revealed, as the patient develops severe anaemia, bone disease, vomiting, high blood pressure, muscle weakness, general tiredness, laboured breathing and ultimately convulsions and loss of consciousness. These changes can be reversed by repeated dialysis or by a successful renal transplant. Like the alimentary tract, the urinary tract is subject to blockage by stone, stricture, prostate enlargement and other troubles requiring surgical relief.

Locomotor system

In the circulatory system and the alimentary system we have already met the unresting muscle of the heart, and the

---

* 'La fixité du milieu interne est la condition de la vie libre.'

smooth muscle which propels food material through the gut. However, the greatest mass of muscle in the body is the voluntary muscle, so-called because it is its contraction under the force of our wills which enables us to carry out voluntary movements. However, these same muscles are also active, without any voluntary effort, in maintaining whatever posture we have adopted; otherwise, we would not be able to stand without thinking about it. The muscles are attached to the bones on which they act by tendons or sinews. (Shakespeare displayed some knowledge of physiology when he made Henry V incite his followers to 'stiffen the sinews, summon up the blood', in preparation for warlike exertion. The muscles tighten the tendons, and the blood flow to muscle greatly increases when the muscles become active.) In actual movement, the joints in the limbs bend and straighten.

Weakness of muscles can arise in general illness (including mental depression, when we 'don't feel like doing anything'); in various diseases of the muscle tissue itself; and when appropriate nervous impulses do not reach the muscle, either because the nerves themselves are diseased, or there is a lesion of the specialized junction between nerve and muscle – the neuromuscular junction or motor end-plate. It is this tissue which is the seat of trouble in myasthenia gravis, in which movements are at first strongly performed, but rapidly become weaker, more so than in normal people, the eye muscles being particularly affected. Although this is an uncommon disease, it is important as a probable example of what are called 'autoimmune diseases', in which the immune system of the body develops antibodies to particular tissues, in this case to the motor end-plate. The appropriate antibodies have been found in patients with this disease, and improvement has been demonstrated in a number of patients following plasma exchange (which removes the antibodies) or removal of the thymus gland (which interferes with the production of antibodies). The symptoms can also be well controlled in many cases with the drug physostigmine. This is an example of how disease can be made better either by attacking the causal mechanism, or by diminishing its effects at a lower level; if medicine could rely only on affecting the prime causes of disease, we would be in a worse case than we are.

Our bones can be affected by violence leading to fracture; also by disease, of which the most common form is known as osteoporosis. With advancing years, more rapidly if activity is diminished by disease or torpor, the protein framework of the bone is diminished, and the bones may collapse, most commonly in the weight-bearing vertebrae of the spinal column. However, by far the most vulnerable segment of the 'moving parts' in the locomotor system is the joints. Arthritis is not often fatal, although some forms of it are associated with general diseases which can lead to death. (For example, in another autoimmune disorder known as disseminated lupus erythematosus, an example of multi-system disease, the joints are indeed affected, but so also are the kidneys, and if death occurs it is likely to be due to renal failure.) Arthritis is, however, a very major cause of chronic pain and consequent ill-health. The two main forms of arthritis are rheumatoid arthritis, which may come on tragically early in life, and cause prolonged illness and crippling, though major deformity can usually be avoided by careful treatment and splinting in the early stages; and osteoarthritis, which comes on later in life, is aggravated by exertion and may become so severe as to require replacement of the affected joint. Hip replacement, which owes so much to the work of John Charnley, is now an effective form of treatment, and some progress is being made with the replacement of other joints.

Perhaps I have described enough systems to give you a picture of what is meant by the term; other systems include the skin, the organs of sense perception (eyes, ears and so on) and the organs of reproduction. The systems I have been talking about so far are fairly clearly defined, both in structure and in function. At one level, they might even be looked on as parts of a machine; but such an outlook is quite misleading, and this becomes obvious as we move on from the level of biological organization represented by such systems to the next level, which is that of the intact single

40

living organism. To help you in making that transition, it is appropriate here to consider a group of systems which are less clearly defined in anatomical terms, but which pervade the entire body in various ways. These are the nervous sytem, the endocrine system, the constituents of the blood and the immune system.

The nervous system

One of the classics of medical literature is *The Integrative Action of the Nervous System*, by Sir Charles Sherrington, who was Professor of Physiology in Liverpool and in Oxford, was a minor poet and lived to an advanced age. Sherrington's writings are a model of lucidity, typified by his Gifford Lectures on 'Man and his nature', which combine science and humanism in exemplary fashion. Integration is a blanket term, to signify that in health our various activities are coordinated, not antagonistic to each other. To give an example at a rather lowly level, we are able to bend our knee not only because the muscles at the back of the thigh which bend the knee (the flexors) are stimulated, but also because those which normally straighten it (the extensors) are made to relax – and this 'inhibition' of the extensors (to use the technical term) is as much a part of the activity as is the stimulation of the flexors. To give another example, if a pin was stuck into your hand, you would draw it away, literally before you had time to think about it – a form of response which is described as 'reflex activity'. But it is also possible to over-ride such a reflex by an effort of the will. Both the coordination of muscle activity and the control over reflex action are accomplished by the activity of higher centres in the nervous system.

In beginning with this important general aspect of the activity of the nervous system, I have of course run ahead of the basics of structure and function. The first great anatomical division of the nervous system is into the *central nervous system* (comprising the brain and spinal cord) and the *peripheral nervous system*, which is the array of nerves that penetrates every tissue of the body. In parallel with these systems is a third system of nervous tissue, known as the sympathetic or *autonomic nervous system*, which is largely responsible for such unconscious activities as regulation of blood flow to different parts of the body, by altering the calibre of blood vessels.

From observation of the effects of injury to different parts of the brain, and also from electrical stimulation of different parts of the brain during surgical operations in man, we know a good deal about which parts of the brain deal with particular functions. The largest part of the brain, the cerebrum, consists of two lobes, right and left. For some unknown reason (unknown to me at least) most of the tracts that bring information from the body to the brain, and convey 'instructions' from the brain to the body, cross from one side to the other on the way up to the cerebrum, so that for a right-handed person, it is the left lobe of the cerebrum which is dominant, and conversely for a left-handed person. The part of the brain dealing with vision lies far back in the cerebrum on both sides, and in a person who has lost the sight of both eyes, a pattern of light can be achieved by stimulation of suitably placed electrodes. Centres for hearing are at the sides of the cerebrum; motor activity and sensory perception are also localized to specific areas of the outer part of the cerebrum, known as the cortex. There are also, however, large areas of brain, towards the front of the cerebrum, whose function is uncertain, but which seem to have some influence on mood, justifying at one time the operation of leucotomy, which cut off these areas from their connection with other parts of the brain and sometimes benefited patients who were depressed. Fortunately, with the advent of pharmaceutical agents for the treatment of depression, this operation is seldom, if ever, performed.

Beneath the cerebrum, and towards the back of the head, is another part of the brain, the cerebellum, which is largely concerned with the maintenance of body posture, a largely unconscious activity. Like other proper activities, this depends on good information, and there is a constant stream of messages telling the brain, and particularly the cerebellum, where the different parts of the body are. Posture is then maintained or altered, as the case may be, by varying the tension in the various muscle groups.

Between the upper parts of the brain and the spinal cord we have the brain stem, comprising the mid-brain and the medulla. The long tracts, both sensory and motor, connecting the body with the cerebrum and cerebellum, obviously must pass through the brain stem, and are vulnerable to damage at this level. Even more critical, however, is the presence in the brain stem of 'centres', ordered collections of nerve cells which maintain the vital functions of breathing and circulation, and which determine our degree of arousal at particular times.

Before saying a little about the spinal cord and the peripheral nerves, let me stress that I have given only the sketchiest account of the relation between structure and function in the brain. The doctor, and particularly the neurologist, has to study these matters in very great detail. At the clinical level, a lesion may involve a group of nerve cells, or may interrupt a nervous pathway or tract; irrespective of the nature of the damage, it is important to discover its situation, and this may in turn give a clue to the nature of the process, or even open up a possibility of surgical treatment. This process of localization of a nervous lesion is based on an extensive series of clinical tests, some of which are familiar, such as the knee-jerk, while others are more specialized, for example detecting whether flashing a light into the eye (visual stimulus) produces an electrical response in the relevant part of the cortex (an evoked potential). Of even wider interest, however, than the localization of neurological disease, is the concept of 'brain death'.

That compressed phrase, brain death, calls for a little explanation. In almost all circumstances it is possible, and usually quite simple, to tell whether a person is dead or alive. But there are exceptions, of which the most relevant at the moment is the situation when a person has had a severe head injury, of which perhaps the most common cause in young people is a traffic accident. Following this, the victim has lost consciousness and may even be unable to breathe on his own account, so that he is now on a respirator, with the aid of which he has a normal pink colour and his heart is beating strongly. Although it is sadly uncommon, people in such a situation may make a gradual recovery, and may even regain their full faculties, though probably carrying a psychological scar for the rest of their lives. On the other hand, the great majority of them gradually deteriorate over a few days or weeks, which is a period of great distress for their family and friends. There is a still more difficult situation, exemplified by the Karen Quinlan case in the USA,★ where the respiratory centre recovers, so that the patient is no longer dependent on a respirator but still remains deeply unconscious. That particular situation is extremely rare, but alas this makes it no easier to deal with in the individual case. At a practical level, the really important distinction to be made is between the first two cases – on the one hand, the person who can recover, however slowly, and is thus clearly 'alive'; and on the other hand, the person who cannot recover, and must thus be presumed 'dead', even though the heart is still beating and respiration is artificially maintained.

Over the years, neurologists and others have developed criteria for 'brain stem death', often contracted to 'brain death', a situation in which the vital centres of the brain stem have been irretrievably damaged by injury or disease. The conditions for making this judgement include a careful analysis of the situation causing the loss of brain stem function, with special reference to whether it could be reversed; ruling out any possibility of the patient's having taken drugs that can lead to coma; absence of particular reflexes whose presence would point to residual brain stem function (these indicators include lack of response of the pupils to light, and failure to choke when tubes are passed into the air-way); and complete failure to breathe spontaneously. Only after a positive result to all these tests (not

★ In 1976, the New Jersey supreme court authorized 'switching off' life-support systems in a 21-year old woman who had been unconscious for a long time. However, she then remained alive, still unconscious, until she died some years later.

just one or two of them) can a patient be considered dead.

A British television programme in October 1980 called these concepts into question, as of course there is a perfect right to do. It was suggested that patients satisfying the accepted criteria for brain death might in fact recover; and that a diagnosis of brain stem death could not be made without making tracings of the electrical activity of the brain (the electroencephalogram). However, the cases brought in support of the possibility of recovery from alleged brain death were all observed in the USA, and none of them would have satisfied the criteria of brain death used in the UK; some of the patients, for example, had taken soporific drugs, which are capable of suspending brain stem function for many hours, until their effects wear off. On the other hand, the EEG, as usually performed, is an indication of the function of the cerebrum, and not of the brain stem.

One good effect came from the programme; a revised code now requires the critical tests to be performed on at least two occasions, which greatly lessens the chance of human error. On the other hand, the programme caused considerable alarm that people might be taken off respirators when they were 'not really dead', and it had a repercussion on the number of kidneys available for transplantation. However, the worst effect of the programme was not on renal transplantation, but on the longer period of anxiety imposed on relatives of irretrievably injured patients, while the matter was being further examined. To date, no case of recovery has been reported in any patient who fully satisfied the criteria for brain death. It would be ludicrous to say that no such patient could ever recover, but the strong likelihood is that such an event would point to human error in the performance and assessment of the tests, rather than to error in the principles underlying them.

I have digressed on to the emotive subject of brain death here to illustrate the importance of thorough knowledge and deep objectivity in making statements on health matters; it is not a job for those whose skills are limited to communication.

Coming now to the *spinal cord*, this is the great channel

through which nervous impulses pass down from the brain to the peripheral nerves, which can then cause muscles to contract and initiate other activities of the body. It also carries impulses in the other direction, conveying information from the body to the brain. Although these are generally called *sensory impulses*, which might imply conscious sensation, the great majority of them are acted on by the brain without ever reaching consciousness. If it were not so, our thoughts would be hopelessly confused by the mass of entering stimuli. The nerve fibres carrying these impulses up and down are not scattered at random, but are arranged in definite bundles, known as *tracts*. The main tracts carrying motor impulses to the muscles lie at the sides of the spinal cord. At the front of the spinal cord are tracts conveying various sensations – touch, pain, heat and cold; and at the back of the spinal cord are the tracts conveying information about the position of different parts of the body, information of which we are unconscious unless we particularly think about it, but which is necessary all the time both for the maintenance of posture and for the toning of muscular movement. If you think of an expert pianist, playing a lively, scherzo passage, you can imagine the complexity to which this information system can be trained.

Besides channelling impulses to and from the brain, the spinal cord has a dumb life of its own, underlying the kinds of reflex activity which have already been mentioned, such as withdrawing a limb in response to a painful stimulus. The independence of this type of activity is well shown by its persistence in the victims of tragic accidents which sever the spinal cord, so that they become totally paralysed and also incapable of sensation below the injury to the cord. Should they be exposed to a normally painful stimulus, they withdraw the limb, even though they do not feel the pain.

The spinal cord carries a relic of the segmental stage of evolution, not by being divided itself into segments, but because the nerves which leave or enter it do so in just over 60 bundles. Those towards the back, known as *dorsal roots*, carry mainly sensory impulses; while those towards the front, the *ventral roots*, carry mainly motor impulses.

Although there is this segregation of function just as they approach the spinal cord, the *peripheral nerves* are mainly mixed, in the sense that they contain both sensory and motor fibres. It is only when they approach their respective end-organs that motor and sensory fibres again separate, the motor to the end-plates in muscles, the sensory to a variety of end-organs associated with the different types of sensation.

The transmission of nervous impulses involves complicated shifts of ions, generating electrical currents, and constituting an important field of physiological study. I have only been describing nervous activity at a gross level, although you may still think it sufficiently complex! It is a system of great intricacy – but it works.

The endocrine system

Whereas the concept of a 'nervous system' is both familiar and of long standing, going back to antiquity, the idea of an endocrine system is less familiar, and the concept itself is less than a hundred years old. We need not look far for the general reasons for the comparatively late recognition of this important system. Anatomically, the nervous system includes large structures such as the brain, spinal cord and the larger nerves. The organs on which the endocrine system is based, however, are multiple, many of them are very small and until recently their function was quite obscure. We are all conscious of many of the activities of the nervous system through pain and the special senses; the endocrine system operates as a rule below the conscious level. Even when diseases of endocrine organs proved fatal, the mechanisms were unknown. For example, Jane Austen almost certainly died because her adrenal glands were destroyed by tuberculous infection, producing one form of Addison's disease; she could now be kept in good health, though not strictly speaking 'cured', by a combination of anti-tuberculous treatment and replacement of the substances normally secreted by healthy adrenal glands.

The comparatively recent recognition of the endocrine system was not due to its lack of importance, but to the lack both of appropriate methods for studying it, and even more of the unifying concept that the integration of bodily function is achieved not only by nervous impulses, as I have just been trying to describe, but also by 'messenger substances' or *hormones* elaborated in a system of glands and carried in the bloodstream to important end-organs whose activity they stimulate. A very large number of hormones are now known, and I shall mention here only those of recognized major importance so far (this note of caution is justified, as new hormones from unsuspected sites such as the gut are frequently being discovered). What we may loosely call well-established hormones are thyroxin, derived from the thyroid gland; insulin from the pancreas; cortisol and adrenalin from the adrenal cortex and medulla; and of course the hormones from the gonads ('sex glands'), such as oestrogen, progesterone and testosterone.

Since hormones are chemical substances, it is not surprising that many of their effects are chemical, influencing the many chemical processes in the body, which are collectively known as 'metabolism'. Thyroxin, for example, stimulates metabolism and insulin allows a major metabolic fuel, glucose, to enter the cells where it can be used. Endocrinology and biochemistry have developed hand in hand, and make up one of the most active fields in current medical research. I shall try here to give some examples to bring out a few principles of endocrine activity.

Many of the processes in which endocrine activity is involved exemplify the principle known as 'negative feedback'. To give a specific example, the concentration of glucose in the blood has to be kept within limits. If it falls too low, the victim feels faint, sweats and may even go into a fatal coma; if it goes too high, the symptoms of diabetes arise, with thirst and various complications, which again may include coma. In health, a rise in blood sugar such as may occur after eating sweets stimulates the appropriate cells in the pancreas to secrete insulin, which then causes a lowering of the blood sugar. On the other hand, when the blood sugar falls for any reason, such as fasting, the secretion of insulin is shut off. It is this type of regulation, where the release of a regulating substance is prompted by a perceived need for its action, which is common to many endocrine processes.

A second point of interest, not perhaps a 'principle', is the way in which so much of our knowledge of the endocrine system derives from diseases that had been recognized long before the concept of an endocrine system had taken shape. For example, the clinical effects of an excess of thyroid hormone were recognized, in the form of exophthalmic goitre or Graves's disease, long before the existence of such substances was suspected. Particularly important in the development of modern medicine was the discovery of insulin by Banting and Best in Toronto in 1922. As a disease, diabetes was known to the Greeks, with its salient features of thirst, copious amounts of sweet-tasting urine and often a fatal ending. In the seventeenth century, Thomas Willis of Oxford clearly distinguished it from another form of diabetes (diabetes insipidus) in which the thirst and outpouring of urine are due not to sugar in the urine, but to lack of a hormone derived from the pituitary gland which enables the kidneys to produce a concentrated urine. In the absence of this 'antidiuretic hormone', the kidneys produce large amounts of dilute urine, and the thirsty patient superficially resembles a sufferer from 'true' diabetes – 'sugar diabetes' or 'diabetes mellitus'. The next step came in the nineteenth century, when it was observed by two German scientists, von Mering and Minkowski, that dogs from which the pancreas has been removed developed diabetes.

By the early years of this century, the concept of endocrine regulation of metabolism was well established, and the search was on for a substance of pancreatic origin which could lower the blood sugar. A practical difficulty was that the pancreas not only makes insulin, but also a digestive enzyme, trypsin, which destroys insulin. Macleod, Banting, Best and Collip all contributed to overcoming this difficulty, at least partially; and the development of insulin as a practical agent of treatment also owed much to the pharmaceutical firm of Lilly. Even if the discovery of insulin was ushered in by a certain amount of good fortune, and later tarnished by disputes over priority, Best particularly shows the scientific virtues of perseverance and a prepared mind; and nothing can obscure the great importance of a discovery which showed that the application of physiological knowledge could produce an effective cure of an important disease. In fact, 'cure' is not strictly correct, since the diabetic person still cannot produce adequate amounts of insulin; but the important thing is that patients can be kept alive for many years who would have died in a few months before 1922.

Of course, discovery did not cease in 1922. We now know much more about different types of diabetes, and the latest development so far is the production of human-type insulin by genetic manipulation of bacteria, which can be used in patients who have become allergic to insulin prepared from cattle or pigs.

This story, which I have given in barest summary, illustrates the contributions made to the tapestry of medical knowledge by the observation of disease states, the use of animal experiments, the application of physiological and biochemical techniques, the role of the pharmaceutical industry in translating laboratory discovery into practical treatment, and most recently, the impact of molecular biology.

By describing them separately, as of course I have to do, I may have given the impression that nervous and hormonal regulation are independent of each other. This is not so, since there is a region in the brain known as the hypothalamus which contains groups of nerve cells which to some extent modulate the activity of the endocrine system by producing 'releasing hormones' which travel down to the pituitary gland, situated just below the hypothalamus, and stimulate this gland to produce hormones which in turn stimulate distant endocrine glands. For example, 'thyrotrophin releasing hormone' stimulates the pituitary to secrete 'thyrotrophin', which then stimulates the thyroid gland to secrete its hormone.

The blood

Goethe makes Mephistopheles say, 'Blut ist ein ganz besonderes Saft', a devilish utterance which might be very loosely rendered as 'Blood is pretty special stuff'. This is indeed so, if we consider the variety of activities within the body for which blood is the necessary medium of transport. Its role in the transfer of oxygen and carbon dioxide between the lungs and the tissues has already been mentioned, and also the hormones which it carries; but it also carries nutrients of many kinds to the tissues, and conveys from them waste products, for disposal by the lungs in the case of carbon dioxide, and by the kidneys and liver in the case of dissolved solids. Many of these transport functions are carried out by the fluid part of the blood, known as the *plasma*, which when separated from the cells of the blood is a clear yellowish fluid, containing proteins, fats and carbohydrates and a great variety of other substances. The walls of the capillaries within which the blood flows through the tissues are thin, and allow salts and water to pass freely through them. It follows that some force must be preventing the plasma from seeping away into the tissues; this force is mainly what is called the 'osmotic attraction' of the proteins in plasma.

The capillary walls do not allow the passage of large molecules, of which the proteins are the most important, and particularly the *albumin* part of the protein, which occurs in a concentration of around 5 g per 100 ml. In some diseases of the liver and kidneys albumin is not formed in adequate amount, or it escapes in the urine when the capillaries of the kidney are damaged, and made abnormally permeable to protein. When the albumin is seriously depleted in either of these ways, salt and water escape into the tissues, which become swollen with fluid, a condition known as 'oedema'. This often affects the legs, under the influence of gravity, and there it can be recognized if a finger is pressed firmly into the swollen area, which is quite painless unless the tissue has become inflamed. Since the fluid is loosely present in the tissues, it can be moved away, and a small depression forms, which fills up again slowly after the finger applying the pressure has been removed. This somewhat dramatic phenomenon is known as 'pitting oedema'; it is still fairly common, but is now more easily controlled since the arrival of powerful 'diuretic' agents, which can remove fluid from the body. In addition to albumin, the blood contains another class of proteins, the *globulins*, which form part of the immune system, of which more later.

The solid constituents of the blood are the red cells, white cells and platelets, which together make up just under half the volume of the blood. As their name might well imply, the *red cells* give the blood its characteristic colour. In each cubic millimetre of blood, the equivalent of a tiny drop, there are five million of them. Unlike most cells of the body, they have no nucleus, but they are packed with a substance *haemoglobin*, an iron-containing pigment which has the vital property of combining very easily with oxygen in the lungs, and parting with it in the tissues. It is bright red when fully saturated with oxygen, and becomes somewhat blue, in noblemen and commoners alike, when it loses oxygen. In the so-called white races, the skin owes its pink colour to well-oxygenated haemoglobin. When someone is anaemic, from blood loss or from faulty formation of blood, it is the lowered level of haemoglobin which causes the pale colour. Also, when people 'go blue with cold', this is because the circulation to the skin is greatly reduced in order to conserve heat, and the relatively stagnant blood in the skin loses its oxygen sufficiently to impart a blue colour to the skin. Unfortunately, the affinity of haemoglobin for gases extends to carbon monoxide, which can even displace oxygen; so the essence of poisoning by exhaust gases is oxygen deprivation through its displacement on the haemo-globin carrier by carbon monoxide. Carboxy-haemoglobin, as the compound is called, is still bright pink, but is useless to the tissues.

Having mentioned that the condition known as anaemia can be due either to blood loss or to faulty formation of red cells, I shall introduce here another general concept of considerable value in practical medicine, the idea of what is called a *syndrome*. This is a grouping of abnormal features which are sufficiently characteristic to be readily recognizable by a trained observer, or even by the patient but which can be brought about in a variety of ways. The practical value of this is that it may be possible to take steps to relieve the patient's discomfort, and with it his anxiety, even before the underlying cause of the condition has been established. It is easier to exemplify a syndrome than to define it and, conveniently for us, anaemis is a particularly good example of a clear-cut state that may, however, be caused in quite a number of different ways. Let me then first of all describe the characteristic features by which a patient with anaemia can be recognized and then illustrate the considerable variety of mechanisms by which anaemia may be brought about.

The recognition of anaemia
The ease with which anaemia can be recognized naturally varies with its severity. Pallor, for example, may be obvious at a glance, but when the anaemia is slight, pallor may have to be looked for. The exposed areas of the skin may not show pallor even when anaemia is quite definite; so we look for it on the palms of the hands, or the inner surface of the lower eyelid. But if there is any doubt in the matter, the best thing is actually to take a blood sample and measure both the amount of haemoglobin in the blood and also the number of red cells. This will not only confirm or disprove the presence of anaemia, but will give a measure of its severity, and also a lead to some possible causes. This advice would be rejected by those who believe that the last ounce of information must be extracted by clinical methods before any investigation is done; but I believe that once a clear problem has been defined, in this case 'Is the patient anaemic?', it is justifiable to take the short-cut of investigation, which can give a clear-cut quantitative answer, while the best clinical evidence on this point may lead only to a surmise.

Having unburdened myself of this heresy, let me consider

the case of the patient, probably an unobservant man, who fails to notice that he is going pale. What will he complain of? The most likely answer is breathlessness, which the doctor may translate to himself as 'dyspnoea', which is Greek for distressed or uncomfortable breathing. This is of course a very common symptom. It may be of purely nervous origin, or due to disease of the heart or lungs; and we can all experience it by taking strenuous exertion. But in the anaemic patient the breathlessness has the particular characteristic that it is absent so long as he is resting, but appears, not on severe exertion, but on such slight exertion as would cause no difficulty to a normal person. Our shorthand, perhaps rather cumbrously, for this state of affairs is 'exertional dyspnoea'.

When the oxygen carrying capacity of the blood is impaired by anaemia, some compensation may be achieved by increasing the amount of blood circulating through the tissues. This implies an increase in the activity of the heart, to an extent which may make the patient aware of it, and complain of palpitation. Feeling the pulse may show a rapid action of the heart, but as a rule the heart beat remains regular. Depending on the degree of anaemia, and also on the personality of the patient, palpitation may be experienced only on exertion, or it may even occur at rest. There are of course other causes of palpitation, some of which are associated with irregularity of the heart beat.

Taken separately, pallor, breathlessness and palpitation each have several possible causes other than anaemia. But when they occur together, they furnish a strong probability (not a certainty – certainties are rare in medicine) that the patient is anaemic. Conversely, individual patients with anaemia may have other features, such as sore tongue, brittle nails, indigestion and bleeding, which are related more to the cause of the anaemia than to its mere presence.

Let us suppose that anaemia has been suspected on clinical grounds, and its presence confirmed by a blood count. An emergency measure is potentially available in the shape of a transfusion of compatible blood; but it rarely has to be taken, except when there is obvious rapid blood loss or where there has been gross delay in detecting the anaemia. But the patient can be told that he is anaemic, and that steps will be taken to discover the cause. This will often allay the anxiety which may account for at least a part of his distress, and that is no mean gain. But matters cannot rest there, until a cause has been discovered and if possible treated. This may be a simple matter, or it may demand complex haematological study. Here I can only indicate some of the main possible causes.

Some causes of anaemia

A scarcity of haemoglobin, which is what anaemia is, may result either because red cells are being lost from the body or, less commonly, because they are being destroyed at an abnormal rate within it; or because red cells are not being formed in adequate amount.

Sudden severe haemorrhage produces a state of surgical shock which overshadows the anaemia which it also produces. The requirement here is to arrest the bleeding and to restore by transfusion not only the haemoglobin, but also the volume of circulating blood. It is the less obvious forms of slow bleeding, such as may occur from a tumour of the stomach or bowel, which may lead to anaemia. In any obscure anaemia the stools should be inspected for visible blood, and clinical tests done for 'occult blood', i.e. blood or its products which are not visible, but are still capable over time of leading to anaemia. If this proves positive, a search for the tumour can be made by X-rays or by direct vision through an endoscope – not forgetting direct examination of the back passage by a finger.

Red cells go bumping round the narrow capillaries many times in their short life of about three months, and in health they are adequately replaced by new red cell formation. The process of red cell destruction is known as 'haemolysis' and there is a group of conditions known as the *haemolytic anaemias* in which destruction is abnormally rapid, to an extent that formation of new red cells in the red bone-marrow cannot keep pace with it, even though the bone-marrow is maximally stimulated to do so, and indeed becomes greatly enlarged at the expense of the fatty bone-marrow. The life-span of red cells can be measured by labelling some of the patient's own cells with a radioactive isotope of chromium, re-injecting them, and measuring the rate of disappearance of radioactivity. When a reduced lifespan of red cells has been demonstrated, further tests are needed to decide whether there is some weakness of the red cells themselves, or whether there are antibodies in the plasma which are destroying them.

In these forms of anaemia (blood loss and haemolysis), the remaining red cells contain about a normal amount of haemoglobin per cell. But in some types of anaemia due to inadequate formation of red cells the situation is different, and a comparison between haemoglobin content and red cell number in the blood may give a clue to the nature of the anaemia. For example, in the form of anaemia due to insufficient iron in the body, iron being a constituent of haemoglobin, not only is the total amount of haemoglobin reduced, but the amount is reduced in each red cell, there being no defect in the actual formation of the red cell substance, but only failure to supply them with the normal amount of haemoglobin. On the other hand, in 'pernicious anaemia' the defect is in the development of the red cells themselves, and each one has its normal complement of haemoglobin, or even more. It is the number of red cells which is greatly reduced.

In considering the possible cause of any condition, weight should be given to the relative prevalence of the different possibilities in the particular situation. In this country, the most likely causes of anaemia might be iron deficiency and chronic loss of blood; whereas in the tropics the most likely causes might be malaria or hookworm infestation.

To return to our discussion of the composition of the blood, the remaining components are the white cells and platelets. The white cells are few in comparison with the red cells, being normally under 10,000 per cubic millimetre. They are nucleated cells, the majority of them having a lobed nucleus, and being capable of destroying bacteria – these are the 'phagocytes' which were 'stimulated' in Shaw's play 'The Doctor's Dilemma'. There are also cells with round nuclei, smaller in number but of great importance in the immune system of the body, known as lymphocytes and macrophages.

The platelets are much smaller than the cells of the blood and their main role is in limiting the effects of injury to blood vessels. When the inner lining of a blood vessel is damaged, platelets accumulate over it. Some of them break up, and this starts the complex sequence of reactions which causes blood to clot, thereby sealing up the damage to the vessel more firmly than the original platelet plug could do. Minor damage to small blood vessels is probably going on all the time, without becoming apparent; but when there is a deficiency of platelets small defects in vessels are not repaired, and serious, even fatal, bleeding can occur in internal organs, as well as more obviously in the skin.

The immune system

This is the collective term given to the various systems of defence which the body has at its disposal, to protect it against potentially harmful substances which may gain access to it. The 'substances' involved include not only large, organic molecules, but also organisms, which include parasites, bacteria and viruses. Throughout our lives we are exposed to such substances and agents; those of them which provoke an *immune response* from one or other component of the immune system are described as *antigens*, with the adjective *antigenic*. (Another term which has been used is 'allergens', but the term 'allergy', from which this is derived, has become so widely used as to weaken its original application.)

The immune response has two major components, each of them somewhat complex, known as the *cellular response* and the *humoral response*. In outline, the cellular response deploys cells with the capacity to kill foreign cells, or to 'swallow' and neutralize foreign particles, a process known as 'phagocytosis'. The humoral response initially also involves cells, but now in the preparation of members of a class of protein known as *globulins* which pass into the blood and body fluids (hence the term 'humoral', which just means 'in the body fluid'). These then act as *antibodies*, combining with the antigens, and protecting the body in various ways from their harmful effects. Not too surprisingly, the cellular and humoral responses often act in concert; a harmful bacterium may provoke the formation of a specific antibody to it, which may then become attached to particular areas of the bacterial surface, which it damages so that the bacterium readily becomes a prey to phagocytic cells.

The immune system is extremely complex, justifying one of the most rapidly developing branches of medical science, that of *immunology*. Although the exasperated student may at times think the opposite, natural processes are not often complicated without reason; the complexity of the immune system is a necessary consequence of its versatility and specificity. It has to be versatile, in view of the number and diversity of the antigens with which it may be called upon to deal; and it has to be specific, in order that the response may be sharp and targeted to the particular antigen, not diffuse and damaging to normal tissue. These ends are achieved by the performance of a remarkable group of cells, the lymphocytes, which lie at the root of both cellular and humoral immunity. One class of lymphocytes, known as the T lymphocytes because they were derived originally from primitive cells in the thymus gland, are responsible for cell-mediated immunity. Another class, the B lymphocytes, are not thymus dependent; they can produce specific antibodies to a very wide range of antigens. The mechanisms whereby these things happen are beyond our present scope; but you may perhaps be curious to know how one type of cell can cope with an almost limitless number of potential antigens. It would clearly be wasteful for an Eskimo to be in a state of constant active readiness to face the malarial parasite, and we may take the view that the specific response is initiated only when a particular antigen comes along. Once an antigen has been encountered however, even if it subsequently dis-appears, a trace seems to remain, and a second exposure to the same antigen, but not to another, evokes a prompter and stronger response. We may therefore have within us a kind of library of memory of previously encountered antigens, in the shape of just a few lymphocytes sensitized to one particular antigen; if it reappears, the appropriate lympho-cytes are stimulated both to multiply and to become active in producing antibody.

A healthy immune system can be manipulated to give protection against threatened disease. The oldest practical application of this was Edward Jenner's vaccination against smallpox; and immunization of infants and children against the commoner infectious diseases is now commonplace. And of course we owe our recovery from many illnesses to the natural development of an immune reaction to the relevant agent.

The immune system takes time to develop its full potential, and for the first few months of life the infant derives some of its immunity from maternal antibodies which have crossed the placenta. At the other end of life, immune responses may become somewhat imperfect, and old people are more vulnerable to infection and possibly also to tumours on this account.

A prerequisite of the immune response is the recognition of an antigen as being 'foreign' to the body. This recognition is imperfect or even absent in the fetus, and foreign material may be tolerated which would be rejected in later life. Transplantation of tissues and organs would be much easier if we could find some way of blunting this recognition of 'foreignness' in adult life; but as things are, we have to fall back on blunting the immune response itself by *immuno-suppressive drugs*. In an oblique way, the use of such drugs indicates the importance of the immune response, as patients so treated are very vulnerable to infections. Apart from the use of drugs, there are some rare congenital conditions in which either the cellular or the humoral response, or even both, are absent or imperfect; such patients are vulnerable, and have a poor life expectancy, though the lack of a humoral response can be coped with by giving immune globulin derived from the blood of healthy donors. The importance of the immune response is also clearly shown, if only by default, in patients with the dangerous acquired immune deficiency syndrome (AIDS).

There are also instances, even apart from the rejection of transplants, where the normally beneficial immune response can cause trouble. Some of us react, it would seem excessively, to foreign material around us, such as pollen, flour etc., and develop hay fever, asthma or eczema. An interesting example of a more concealed abnormal reaction is found in the condition known as coeliac disease or steatorrhoea, where the cells of the small bowel are abnormally sensitive to the protein of wheat and other cereals; abnormal sensitivity to gluten impairs the absorptive power of the gut, and this becomes most obvious in relation to the absorption of fats, the patient passing large, pale, offensive fatty stools. It should be noted that, while distinctly troublesome, these are still specific reactions to specific antigens and the concept of a general immune response to the whole environment, suggested by the term 'total allergy syndrome' is based on allegation rather than on rigid proof. Another example of what may loosely be called 'immunological perversity' is afforded by the autoimmune diseases, in which normal body proteins come to be perceived as 'foreign' and become the object of attack; examples are some forms of thyroid disease, haemolytic anaemia and, possibly, pernicious anaemia.

OUTLINE OF GENERAL PATHOLOGY

Early in this chapter, I introduced the concept of levels of biological organization, and so far we have considered the physico-chemical level, the subcellular and cellular levels and, at somewhat greater length, though not in any real detail, the level of the physiological system. The two major regulating systems, nervous or neural, and endocrine, could now serve as a link between these 'lower' levels and the 'higher' levels represented by the whole man and by society. The psychological and societal levels were indeed mentioned towards the end of Chapter 2, and we will return to them in later sections of the book. But I want now to complete my brief attempt to answer the impossible question 'What is disease?' by some discussion of certain processes of disease which can affect different levels of organization and different physiological systems. These come under the heading of 'general pathology'. By definition, they are not part of normal healthy life, but are specific 'disease mechanisms'.

I have already discussed, in specific contexts, a few of the many ways in which the body or its parts can react to damaging agents. I will now deal with the types of agent that can be harmful to the body and with some of the reactions to them which can be manifest in any part of the body, without respect to any particular physiological system.

Damaging agents

I outlined earlier the mechanisms underlying those diseases which have a genetic basis, and this outline should now be complemented by an indication of the main types of agent which can be responsible for diseases that are not genetically determined. *Physical* causes of disease include mechanical injury, thermal or electrical injury, and injury due to ionizing radiation; to these might be added physical changes internal to the body, such as blockage of blood vessels and the pressure or blockage effects arising from the growth of tumours. *Chemical* causes of disease include a vast range of poisonous substances; disturbances of the metabolic reactions within the body; and faulty nutrition, including deprivation of food and fluid, deficiency of proteins and vitamins in the diet and also excesses of fat and carbohydrates leading to obesity. *Infection* with micro-organisms (bacteria or viruses) is a frequent cause of both acute and chronic disease. *Infestation* with parasites can affect the skin (scabies and pediculosis), the gut (tapeworms and hookworm) and other internal organs (filariasis, 'sleeping sickness' (trypanosomiasis) and malaria). Disturbances of the *immune system* are an important cause of general disease, the most

61

topical example being the acquired immune deficiency syndrome (AIDS). The weakening of the immune defences of the body in old age is relevant to a poor response to infections, and also very possibly to the increased prevalence of tumours in the elderly. The Australian immunologist MacFarlane Burnet has championed the view that potential transformation of cells towards malignancy may be quite common, but the effective surveillance by the immune system prevents them from developing into full-blown tumours, by recognizing the transformed cells as 'foreign' and then destroying them. Of course, another category of disease, including asthma and eczema, represents an exaggerated response of the immune system to a variety of allergens. Finally, much disease is caused or aggravated by *psychological* reactions to the manifold stresses of life, or by adverse *social* circumstances.

General reactions of tissues

These occur in great variety, including the complex processes of *wound healing*; the growth of tissues in response to increased demand, known as *hypertrophy*, and perhaps most visible in the contrast between the muscles of the athlete and the wasted limbs of a bed-ridden patient; the various reactions mounted by the body against infection and infestation. Two general reactions, however, are of overwhelming importance, one being a protective mechanism, at least in moderation – *inflammation* – the other essentially destructive and even lethal – *tumour formation*.

Inflammation

The characteristic appearances of inflamed superficial tissue were well described by Celsus at the beginning of the Christian era, as 'calor, rubor, tumor et dolor' (heat, redness, swelling and pain). These classic signs are associated with impairment of function of the affected tissue or part of the body – for instance, the rather striking way in which an injured limb is held motionless. Strictly speaking, these are the signs of 'acute' inflammation, the early response to injury or to damaging agents, physical, chemical or biological; when the stimulus is less intense, but also more prolonged, the body's response is different, constituting a state of 'chronic' inflammation, characterized by formation of what is called *granulation tissue*, which later becomes fibrous, and may ultimately lead to a scar, such as may be visible on the surface of the body following an injury but may also be the end-stage of damage to internal organs. We shall not consider chronic inflammation further, but acute inflammation is such a common and important response to a great variety of damaging agents that the main processes involved should at least be mentioned.

Soon after injury or damage, there is a great increase in the flow of blood through the affected tissue or part of the body. This is achieved by widening of the small arteries (arterioles) carrying blood to the tissue, and is known as 'active hyperaemia', which is simply a term for a positive increase in blood flow. If one admits the daring possibility that biological reactions may in themselves have a purpose then the purpose of this hyperaemia may be to allow increased access of blood-borne defensive agents, both cellular and humoral (terms explained in my discussion of the immune system), to the affected part; and also, of course, to drain away waste products.

Since the ultimate action takes place largely outside the blood vessels, and since these normally prevent the passage of cells and protein through their walls, there must be some increase in their permeability to allow access of protective cells and protein to the tissue spaces. This escape into the tissues of materials that would normally be retained within the capillaries is known as 'exudation', and the fluid so leaked into the tissues is known as the inflammatory exudate. This process largely accounts for the swelling and pain of inflamed tissue.

As the tissue becomes more congested with exudate, the initially rapid blood flow in the capillaries slows down, and the polymorph leucocytes ('phagocytes') adhere to the walls of the capillaries, and then pass through them into the tissue spaces to take part in the inflammatory response. This emigration of leucocytes brings into play the cellular response to the damaging stimulus.

Underlying these visible changes, there is a complex system or systems of chemical mediators, some of which are enzymes, others components of the complement system, and others simpler substances such as histamine (perhaps most directly known to sufferers from pollen allergy, which can be partly controlled by the anti-histamine agents). These chemical mediators act in sequence, and so to some extent do the cellular components of the inflammatory response. In the acute phase, it is the actively phagocytic *polynuclear leucocytes* which predominate; later, these are largely replaced by *mononuclear cells,* and later still the appearance of *fibroblasts* ushers in the more chronic inflammatory response. In the skin, scarring is as a rule harmless; but in some internal organs, such as the liver or kidney, active tissue may gradually be replaced by fibrous or scar tissue. In the liver this process is known as cirrhosis, whose commonest cause is the consumption of considerable amounts of alcohol over a long period. Fortunately, the most common outcome of acute inflammation is complete resolution – inflammation is something we have all experienced, and yet by and large we live on.

Tumour formation

Troublesome though it may be at its height, there is at least a good side to inflammation; but the same can scarcely be said of tumour formation. The word itself only means a swelling, but in popular usage it often denotes a dangerous, spreading or *malignant* growth, something which should more properly be called a *cancer,* to distinguish it clearly from the many forms of so-called *benign* tumour, which remain localized, although they can sometimes cause trouble, not by spreading through the body, but by local pressure on vessels, nerves or other tissues. We are probably all familiar with benign tumours of the skin, especially in later life, when a variety of nodules and skin tags can appear, not to mention the warts that can occur at any age. Benign tumours in great variety can arise in almost every tissue or situation in the body, but for the present purpose, let me follow popular interest and concern by concentrating on malignant tumours, grouped together as 'cancer'.

Perhaps the first thing to say is that such a grouping together is, at least in one sense, misleading. Cancer is very far from being a single disease, condition or entity. What the various conditions which make up 'cancer' have in common is uncontrolled growth, often coupled with a tendency to 'seed off' into other parts of the body. These characteristics are respectively termed 'local malignancy' and 'disseminated malignancy', or 'metastasis'. The individual varieties of cancer, however, differ very greatly in the type of tissue from which they arise; in the speed or slowness of their growth; in the factors that cause them, so far as these are known; and in the local and general reaction to them, which is an important factor in determining both their natural history and the outcome of treatment. We have indeed a whole constellation of diseases, and to expect a single 'cure for cancer' is unrealistic. That may sound gloomy, but remember that some forms of cancer are already 'curable', in the sense that lifespan is not shortened by them; and in others, particularly the childhood leukaemias, the outlook is vastly better than it was even a decade ago. Of course the challenge of many other forms of cancer remains, and my message is that we can legitimately expect piecemeal improvements in treating specific forms of cancer, but probably not the global breakthrough which we would all of us want. But how happy I would be if some fundamental discovery made me eat these words.

To return to the general characteristics of cancers, I mentioned *uncontrolled growth* and the *liability to spread* both locally and to other parts of the body. Growth as such is of course a cardinal feature of living organisms, both obviously in the procession from babyhood to maturity, and more subtly in the constant process of replacement of outworn cells. We may not have the capacity of the frog to develop a new limb when one has been lost, but if we lose say a part of our liver by accident or by surgery, regeneration of liver tissue takes place approximately to replace the amount which has been lost. We can see how a feedback mechanism could match the amount of tissue replaced to that which had been lost; but it is more of a puzzle why the shape of the original organ should be more or less reproduced. With cancerous tissue, however, the situation is quite different; control is in abeyance, and the cells grow very actively, but without regard to the needs of the body, and even to the invasion and destruction of adjacent tissues. Actively growing cancers lose the structural features of the tissue from which they developed, and they also have a rich blood supply, which makes them liable to haemorrhage. In addition to these local effects, cancerous cells may gain access to the blood stream, the likelihood of this being increased by their rich blood supply; or they may enter the lymphatic system, and spread in that way to neighbouring, or even distant lymph glands. It is even possible for a small cancer to become apparent, not through any local effects, but by the appearance of distant metastases, or secondary deposits. Cancers may also reveal themselves in still more bizarre ways, by affecting the function of nerves in the limbs (an unexplained but well-established happening), or by secreting hormones without regard to the needs of the body. This *inappropriate secretion of hormones* is consistent with the idea that many tissues may contain cells with potential endocrine activity, and as the proper activity of the tissue becomes disorganized by tumour growth, these cells may as it were cut loose, and develop their latent capacity for hormone secretion.

We do not know the 'cause of cancer', but we do know the causes of some cancers, and indeed the diversity of known causes forms part of the evidence against a unitary theory of cancer causation. A general question which might be asked would be whether cancer is something to which we are doomed by our genetic make-up, or something we acquire from exposure to some damaging agent. To this, the misleading short answer would be, 'Mostly the latter'; i.e., so far as we know at present, environmental influences predominate over inherited characteristics as causes of cancers. At the extremes, there are clear-cut instances of cancers 'caused' by inheritance, or by environmental carcinogens (cancer-causing agents). There is a clear-cut pattern of inheritance, as a Mendelian dominant, of rather rare cancers of the large bowel and of the retina of the eye; at the other extreme, exposure to a large variety of organic chemicals (aniline dyes, coal-tar products and so on) has been shown to be the determining agent in a variety of cancers. Much of the most valuable evidence for the importance of environmental agents comes from epidemiological studies, and what may be a very clear message for the health of a population may be confused by exceptions at the level of the individual patient.

To give a concrete example, and one of great practical significance, the epidemiological evidence for an association between cancer of the bronchus and the smoking of cigarettes could scarcely be stronger. It is based not only on comparisons between smoking and non-smoking populations at the same time, but also on the time-course of smoking habits and subsequent experience of bronchial cancer. But there are less common forms of bronchial cancer which are not demonstrably related to smoking; and of course many smokers die not of bronchial cancer, but of something else. These facts, for such they are, are of course given particular prominence by those with an interest in propagating the smoking habit; but when set in context, they are scarcely an argument for smoking. They do, however, lessen the confidence with which, in any particular individual with bronchial cancer, we can say that it was due to smoking.

However, for other common cancers, such as those of the breast, uterus and alimentary tract, the balance between host factors and environmental agents is still less clear-cut. Clustering of cases of say cancer of the stomach within a family does occur, sometimes to a striking degree, but the great majority of patients show no such effect. Of course, host factors need not be limited to inherited factors; I have already mentioned Burnet's view that the waning of the immune response with advancing years may account in part for the increased incidence of cancers in the elderly. This view is supported by the increased incidence of cancer in patients whose immune response has been suppressed either by disease, or by agents given to prevent rejection of a transplanted kidney; but the increased incidence of such cancers is accounted for mainly by tumours arising from lymphoid tissue, and not by other forms of cancer.

Since we cannot as a rule determine our parents, or indeed renew our immunological youth, much attention has quite properly been paid to studying the role of environmental causes of cancer, some of which at least might be avoided, given clear enough evidence, and also sufficient individual and collective will. The major carcinogenic agents to be considered are chemical, physical and viral.

Chemical carcinogens Of the thousands of chemicals known to be capable of inducing tumours, the great majority are organic compounds, the main groups being cyclic hydrocarbons and compound amines; but there are also inorganic carcinogens, most topically asbestos, but also arsenic, beryllium and chromium. The recognition of chemical carcinogenesis goes back a long way; just over 200 years ago the surgeon Percivall Pott recognized the high prevalence of cancer of the scrotum in chimney-sweeps, and related it to soot collecting in the folds of the skin covering the genitalia. (The significance of the observation was enhanced by the rarity of scrotal cancer in the general population.) The practice of sending little boys up chimneys has been discontinued, but other forms of cancer associated with particular occupations continue to be recognized, such as tumours of the bladder in aniline dye workers, of the pleura in asbestos workers, and so on. Chemical carcinogens in all their diversity have this in common, that their effects are gradual, perhaps taking years to produce an actual cancer. The process may be speeded up by other chemicals, which by themselves would not produce cancer, and by susceptibility on the part of the host. On the other hand, cessation of exposure may prevent the appearance of a cancer, and less commonly may allow an established tumour to regress. In some cases, changes can be recognized in tissues before an actual tumour develops, and these pre-cancerous changes may call attention to possible exposure to a cancer-producing agent.

The recognition of cancer-producing properties in compounds already in use is retrospective, and obviously important; but it would clearly be better, in the case of new compounds, to detect carcinogenicity in advance. Because of the latency of the process, however, this testing has to be prolonged, and it also has to be carried out in more than one species. To illustrate this point, suspicion fell on naphthylamine as the particular cause of bladder cancer in aniline dye workers. Tests on several species were negative, but after several years dogs exposed to naphthylamine were found to develop cancers of the bladder similar to those found in the dye workers.

There is considerable altruistic concern about the use of animals, over prolonged periods and in large numbers, to try to rule out the risk of cancer from substances, whether foods or medicines, intended for human consumption; and also from substances to be applied to the human skin. It should also be conceded that, because of species variation, the risk of causing human cancer can never be totally ruled out by animal experiment. Here, however, I must state my own belief that both governments and the general public are well justified in asking for rigorous testing of potential carcinogenic substances. On the other hand, it is not surprising that alternatives to testing for carcinogenicity in animals have been actively sought. One approach of this kind is based on testing for 'mutagenicity' in bacteria. Some strains of bacteria have a potential variability in their genetic make-up, which can lead to detectably different strains of bacteria. It has been observed that this process can be enhanced by various substances which are also known to be carcinogenic. The association between mutagenesis and carcinogenesis is not so close as to make the testing of mutagenic activity an absolute replacement for testing in animals; nevertheless, if a new compound showed strong mutagenic activity, and had no very striking advantages over related compounds, an industrial firm might well hesitate to embark on full-scale testing for carcinogenicity, and would probably not continue development.

Physical agents Cancers due to radioactive products of nuclear fission are a very legitimate cause of public concern; but they have only been relatively recently recognized, and artificially produced radiation is a relatively infrequent cause of cancer, even compared with other physical agents.

Occupational exposures of outdoor workers to sunlight, and the more recent phenomenon of voluntary prolonged exposure on beaches, carry a burden of skin cancers, related to ultra-violet light. Mechanical irritation is a much less common cause of cancer, but there is some association between ill-fitting false teeth and tumours of the mouth. Natives of Kashmir at one time carried braziers with glowing charcoal in front of their bellies, and some developed skin tumours there; but it is uncertain whether this was an effect of heat, or of carcinogenic products of combustion. It is likely, however, that the most important natural physical cause of cancer is the *natural radiation* to which we are all exposed. This includes cosmic radiation from outer space, much of which is screened off by the atmosphere, and terrestrial radiation from radioactive compounds in the earth's crust, which find their way into both the environment and our bodies. Under all ordinary circumstances, natural radiation accounts for over three-quarters of our radiation exposure, the rest coming from medical and industrial applications of radioactivity, and a now diminishing amount from fall-out from the testing of nuclear weapons in the atmosphere.

Natural radiation has no doubt been causing tumours in men and animals from time immemorial; but the knowledge that it could do so had to await our knowledge of radiation and its effects. There have of course been clues, such as the high incidence of cancer in pitch-blende miners, and in girls exposed to thorium in the painting of luminous watches. A few years after the discovery and widespread application of X-rays in medical practice, it was noted that workers developed tumours of the exposed skin. As radiation became more penetrating, tumours of deeper tissues, and particularly of the bone-marrow, began to be noted in patients.

A very specific example was the occurrence of myeloid leukaemia in the children of mothers who had had the dimensions of the bony pelvis established radiologically during pregnancy, a procedure discontinued once its dangers had been recognized, and also because of the decreased prevalence of contracted pelvis now that childhood rickets, once known as the English disease, is a rarity in our native population.

The question naturally arises in peoples' minds, 'Is there any level of radiation below which there is no risk?'. We do not really know for sure, but there has certainly never been any demonstration of a 'threshold', and I personally doubt whether one exists. But this does not of course mean that we must straightway abandon both the medical and the industrial applications of radioactivity; as with other hazards of life, we must minimize them and control them. Military applications are another matter, but the questions they raise are more moral than medical – the medical contribution being to stress the total horror which any full-scale nuclear war would bring to us all.

Let me get out of the para-politics into which I seem to have strayed, by turning to another of nature's Pandora gifts, the viruses.

Viral agents   Viruses are small particles of living matter, less 'structured' even than bacteria, which can cause a wide range of diseases in plants and in animals, including man. Some viruses have the interesting property of existing undetected within the cells of our bodies until we get a mild fever, such as may be due to infection with one of the many viruses that can cause 'the common cold'; at this point the latent virus becomes active, and we see its effects as a 'cold sore'. When the cold passes off, the virus resumes its harmless latency within our cells (the particular virus involved is the herpes simplex virus). It has been known since early in this century that a tumour of chickens could be transmitted by a cell-free filtrate, indicating a viral agent; and similar tumours have been discovered in animals, both solid tumours and the leukaemias.

Viruses that can cause cancer are known as *oncogenic*

71

viruses. It was natural to ask whether oncogenic viruses might be latent in apparently normal human cells, but later be activated to produce cancers. Obviously, transmission of tumours by a filterable agent cannot be tested for in man; and the demonstration of viruses in human tumours does not establish that the virus is the cause. Evidence for a viral cause of some human tumours has indeed been slow in coming; and it must be unlikely that viruses can be responsible for the generality of tumours, especially as some of these have known specific causes such as I described earlier under the heading of chemical and physical agents. Even in such cases, however, the possibility is not excluded that viruses might play some part in the process, not as primary carcinogens, but as sensitizing agents, or 'co-carcinogens'.

The most clearly established human association between a particular virus and a particular form of cancer is that between Epstein–Barr virus (EBV) and Burkitt's lymphoma. To explain these terms, EBV is a common virus world-wide, whose most familiar effect is to cause infectious mononucleosis, or glandular fever; as these names suggest, the fever is associated with an increase in mononuclear cells, and swelling of lymph glands. In most countries, the illness is unpleasant while it lasts but then usually clears up completely, with no long term effects. In East Africa, however, Denis Burkitt discovered that children had an abnormally high frequency of lymphoma – a tumour of lymphoid tissue – and that these tumours contained EBV particles. These could of course have been innocent con-taminants, until it was shown that EBV added to normal human lymphocytes would transform them into cancer cells similar to those found in the tumours.

Preoccupation with rare or exotic diseases is sometimes imputed to academic doctors, so it may be worth noting that study of particular uncommon entities may cast light on important general problems; and that the vital clue in this particular matter came from observations made by a practising surgeon in the tropics. We still do not know the general importance of viruses in causing human cancer, but the possibility is now established.

CONCLUDING REMARKS

As I said at the beginning of this chapter, justification for the use of the terms 'disease' and 'diseases' does not lie in their philosophical validity (for they are interactions, and not substantial entities); it lies rather in their pragmatic value in communication, both directly and at a distance. Understanding of disease can only grow out of some understanding of normal health, and this is looked at in various ways. Life is organized at various levels – the physico-chemical, the cellular, the level of physiological systems, the integration of these into whole organisms, and of these in turn into society. Normal and abnormal functioning can be considered at these various levels; but there are also general processes of disease which call for a degree of independent consideration, including that of the variety of agents which may cause them.

Any one of these topics could be illustrated by a host of specific details, but I have tried to limit myself to the minimum required to clarify a principle. For anyone seeking to know more of these matters, there are ample textbooks of physiology, pathology and medicine available. A glance at any one of these textbooks will show you how much I have omitted from this chapter, but my aim has been not to make you conversant with the knowledge on which modern medicine is based, but merely to give you some indication of its general nature. There have been huge omissions – the properties of parasites, bacteria and viruses; information on the substances and techniques used in medical practice; and virtually the entire realm of psychological abnormality and mental illness. An important, if necessary, omission has been my failure to give any adequate indication, apart from a few scattered hints, of the way in which this body of knowledge has been attained. But I feel it is now time for us to get down to the practicalities of the medical process, as it currently operates at the individual level between doctor and patient.

PART II

The Application of Medical Knowledge to Individual Patients

I hope that the small sample I have been able to give may have shown you the kind of knowledge that would be spread before you on a medical course; I may even have convinced you of its potential value. But of course its value can only be realized if that knowledge is then effectively applied, and the remainder of this book will deal with the applications of medical knowledge. This section describes how medical knowledge can be applied for the benefit of individual patients; in the third part of the book I will consider the more general application of medical knowledge to the health of populations and of society.

It may be helpful to divide the process of applying medical knowledge and skills to the individual patient into three stages. The first is to define the nature and extent of the problem in the particular person (*diagnosis*). The second is to work out a plan of action for dealing with it within the limits of what is possible (there is no entirely satisfactory term for this stage – 'treatment' is too limited and 'management' too authoritarian, but I find *management* marginally the better provided that it is clearly understood that what doctors give is 'advice' and not 'orders', that we are at best 'advisory experts and not autonomous decision-makers'). The third stage is for the doctor to discuss with the patient, and with relatives, his view of the situation, and what he advises should be done (often summarized as *communication*, but again this may be too narrow a term if it is limited to the exchange of words – much of the process is the establishment of a relationship, often largely by non-verbal communication, by look and touch, and securing the relationship by continued interest in the patient's progress).

Before entering into detail, I would emphasize at this stage that these three activities – diagnosis, management and communication – are separated for convenience of discourse; they are neither rigidly successive in time, nor constant in their relative importance. Let me try to justify these two statements, and first that these three stages overlap in time. If there is a way of establishing a diagnosis and implementing a plan of management without in some way communicating with the patient, I have yet to learn it. From the very beginning of the attempt to define the problem, a relationship begins to be formed; and the doctor's estimate of the character of the patient is one component in forming a realistic plan of treatment (equally, it is the patient's estimate of the doctor which largely determines whether he will follow it). One can raise objections to this, such as what happens with a young child, a mentally handicapped person, a deaf patient, or someone who speaks another language and there is no interpreter available? Well, these are real difficulties, but they do not exempt the doctor from conveying in his approach at the very least a desire to help. Even if the problem is both obvious and trivial, like a sprained ankle, the desire to help must be made plain, otherwise the service is incomplete and is the less likely to be acceptable. These sentiments can be criticized as idealistic, or even worse, paternalistic, but I, on the contrary, see them as the essence of good medical practice.

To come to the second point, so obvious that it is often overlooked, there is no fixed order of importance among diagnosis, management and communication. The problems in medical diagnosis range from the very obvious (of which an example has just been given with the sprained ankle) to the virtually insoluble (where some vital piece of knowledge is lacking, or a vital clue has failed to become apparent). Turning to management, this ranges from simple advice right through to complicated schemes of medical treatment or surgical operations of marvellous ingenuity. The ease or difficulty of communication is again very variable, the main factors being the complexity of what has to be communicated, the intelligence of *both* parties, doctor and patient, and the degree of rapport which has been established between them.

These considerations seem to me, at least, to relegate debates on the relative importance of diagnosis and treatment, or communication and management, to the level of verbal pyrotechnics. The simple truth is that they are all important and in the next few chapters we will look at each in detail. For convenience, I have to do this serially; but do not forget that they are all parts of a single process.

4

Diagnosis

From its birthplace in medical jargon, the term 'diagnosis' has escaped into the freedom of general use; but it remains, like 'time' or 'space', easier to understand than to define. I cannot think of any one-word equivalent, so I shall fall back on philosopher Ludwig Wittgenstein's maxim that the meaning of a word is the way in which it is used.* In that sense, diagnosis means 'defining the nature of a medical problem'; 'getting to grips with what is the matter'; or even 'naming the disease', which is closer to the popular sense of the word, although it involves the concept of 'a disease', the philosophic weakness of which I pointed out at the beginning of chapter 3.

What I am trying to do in this chapter is to describe the way in which doctors set about this particular task. The need for 'making a diagnosis' can arise in a number of different ways, and this in turn must affect the nature of the process. For example, there are quite different ways of dealing with routine medical examinations; with requests for particular procedures, such as immunization or even the humble 'certificate', in its infinite variety; with those accidents and emergencies in which the prima facie problem at least is obvious; and with reassessment visits by patients in whom the primary diagnosis has already been established. There is also the very important special case of the care of a woman during pregnancy and childbirth. However, the situation I

* 'Die Bedeutung eines Wortes ist sein Gebrauch in der Sprache.'

particularly want to consider is that in which the majority of practising doctors often find themselves – a man, woman or child notices something which makes them concerned about their health, and they decide to consult their doctor, as a 'patient'. The subsequent interview is generally called a 'consultation', or simply 'a visit to the doctor'; these are better terms than 'examination', which has other meanings, and also over-emphasizes the physical examination, which is only one component of the consultation and not necessarily the most important.

The problem may, of course, be a very obvious one, and the consultation correspondingly short, ending either in reassurance or in simple treatment. At the other extreme the problem may be complex, and the first interview is then merely the prelude to further observation and investigation, which may include admission to hospital. For these reasons, consultations with a general practitioner, a hospital physician* and a surgeon differ in duration, and to some extent in character.

Not surprisingly, my description of the diagnostic process is primarily based on my own experience as a hospital physician, trying to deal with problems in which my help has been sought by a family doctor. Such a consultation takes more time than can usually be afforded by a family doctor, although it is the practice of some doctors to set aside time to see at greater length selected patients who appear to have a particular problem. By the time a patient is referred to a hospital physician, a very considerable degree of selection has already taken place; the potential patient has probably put up with the trouble for a time, hoping that it may go away; he may have talked about it with relatives and friends, and perhaps with a pharmacist, and he has already seen his family doctor. By the time a sufferer from an episode of illness has made his way through these various screens, he may well feel entitled to reasonably thorough

* A general practitioner is sometimes referred to as a 'physician', or even a 'physician and surgeon'; but the term 'physician' is usually applied to a specialist physician with a hospital appointment.

consideration of his problem, and that is what he should get.

The diagnostic process can usefully be divided into three main stages – the taking of a history, the physical examination and often, though not always, a course of investigation. Of these, the first – history-taking – is in general the most important, partly because it constitutes the patient's introduction to the procedure, and also because a careful history may by itself go a very long way towards solving the problem. There is some objective evidence of this, from studies where the physician has written down his provisional opinion at the end of taking the history, and before examining the patient or carrying out any tests. In the great majority of cases, the provisional and the ultimate diagnosis were the same. In stressing the importance of the history, however, we must not relegate physical examination and investigation to unimportance. Either of them may throw up a critical piece of information, unsuspected during the history; also, the history may itself be imperfect, if rapport has not been achieved between the patient and doctor, or if the process is handicapped by deafness, haste or stupidity on either side.

Before coming to the components of history-taking, and even at the risk of repetition, I cannot emphasize too much the heavy responsibility which lies on the doctor to put the patient as much at ease as is possible in the situation. There is a very real disparity between the doctor, a trained professional, in presumably good health, on the one hand, and a patient, however intelligent and cultivated, who is worried about his health and who finds himself in unfamiliar surroundings. At the risk of seeming idealistic and even fanciful, I would say the proper relationship between doctor and patient should in some way resemble that between a host and a guest, with the obligations which that implies. It does not, of course, imply over-elaboration of manner, which can be just as off-putting as brusqueness. Of course some patients, like some guests, may overstay their welcome; most doctors, either instinctively or from practice, develop methods of shortening or concluding an interview within the bounds of courtesy, which should never be transgressed. In making these points, I am anticipating the important subject of communication; but proper communication cannot even begin until rapport has at least begun to be established.

The first step in taking a history is to discover as precisely as possible what is worrying the patient. This is described as 'the presenting symptom', or even the 'complaint'. Of course, in an imperfect world, the presenting symptom may be plural, or even multiple; but since worries, at least to a limited extent, compete for attention, it is usually possible, after a time, to discover what the main concern really is. At this early stage you should note the distinction between a 'symptom' and a 'sign'. A *symptom* denotes something which a patient feels, like a pain, a tingling, or – paradoxically – a loss of sensation in some part of the body, such as happens when a sensory nerve is injured or diseased. A *sign* is something which is either discovered by the doctor, or objectively observed by the patient: for example, the doctor may discover raised blood pressure or signs of anaemia, as described in chapter 3, which the patient may not have noticed; while the patient himself may discover a rash, or discover a lump somewhere. The distinction between symptoms and signs is not absolute – for example, a patient may feel weakness in a limb (symptom) or the doctor may discover it in the course of testing muscle-power (sign); but the distinction has some value, if only to encourage the careful use of language.

The term *complaint* also deserves a little attention. In its everyday use it tends to imply that someone is to blame for what has happened. It is used in this sense when we talk about complaints against doctors or against health authorities, or about 'complaints procedures'. But in the context of taking a history, the term 'complaint' does not necessarily imply blame in any personal sense. Of course, a depressed patient may come, like the prophet Job, to curse his day –

'Let the day perish wherein I was born' – but complaints against the universe are impersonal. Equally, patients do not often view themselves as the authors of their own misfortune and say with Edgar in *King Lear*, 'The gods are just, and of our pleasant vices, Make instruments to plague us'. Again, the use of the word complaint, at least at the beginning of an illness, does not imply blame against the doctor, whatever may happen later if the course of the illness proves disappointing, or if the illness either is or appears to be badly handled – 'badly' often meaning 'unsympathetically' rather than 'incompetently' in objective terms.

Sometimes, the complaint comes bursting forth, but more often, it is left to the doctor to ask questions. I do not believe that many doctors would start by saying to a patient, 'What is wrong with you?', inviting the reply, 'That's for you to discover'. But it is part of the lore of medical schools to warn against that particular way of beginning the interview. Again, I do not greatly like the opening, 'Why have you come to see me?', as it could be taken to imply a less than warm welcome. No, the patient should be greeted in whatever conventional fashion seems appropriate and asked to sit down. Only then should we get down to business, with a neutral question such as 'What have you felt wrong?', or 'What have you noticed that makes you want to see a doctor?'. These are appropriate questions when the patient has been referred for advice about an illness. If you are not sure that this is the situation, it might be safer to say 'How can I help you?'.

The statement of the complaint, when it comes, will naturally and properly be in the patient's own words, but both for the purposes of record, and for expediting the process of diagnosis, it must both be analysed, and also translated into medical terminology. You may well ask why. To take the second of these issues first, the advantage of keeping the record in medical terminology is that it may be easily understood if the patient sees a different doctor in the same or a later episode of illness. The need for analysis of a complaint requires fuller explanation. It makes good sense at least to start with what interests the patient, so that he is well inclined to describe it; but it is difficult for a patient to know what aspects of a symptom are likely to possess medical significance. This can perhaps be best brought out by a specific example. Let us suppose that a patient complains of a cough. He may reasonably wish to emphasize the act of coughing itself, or describe it in detail; whereas a doctor may attach more meaning to the character of the sputum which is brought up, given of course that the coughing is productive of sputum, and not just a dry cough. The presence or absence of pain when the patient coughs is important, but that of course is likely to be mentioned if positive; but the absence of pain is also significant, and may have to be asked for. It is worth remembering that taking a history is not the same as cross-examining a witness in the courts; we are presumed to be on the side of the patient, and not dealing with a hostile witness. It is then quite proper, as it would not be in a court of law, to ask 'leading questions', i.e. those which suggest an answer. For example, if we want to know whether a cough is associated with breathlessness, we do better to ask straight out, rather than to embark on a long series of questions in the form, 'Have you noticed anything else?'. In summary, the analysis of the presenting symptom or complaint should be purposeful and directed, not random and diffuse. An important part of the art of history-taking is to winnow what is essential, and get it into a concise form, but without appearing to be in a hurry.

The nature of the presenting symptom may direct the doctor's attention to a particular physiological system of the body. For example, cough might be associated with disease of the respiratory system, stomach pain with disease of the digestive system, weakness of a limb with disease of the nervous system, or of the muscles themselves, and so on. Leads of this kind should be followed up, by asking about other possible symptoms connected with the suspect physiological system; and additional symptoms so discovered should in turn be subjected to further analysis. Suppose, for example, that our patient with cough is also found, on enquiry, to suffer from breathlessness. We must now discover by further questioning whether this is present all the time, or only on exertion; whether it is associated with wheezing; or if it only happens at night, on lying down. By following this kind of inquiry, we may strengthen the impression that we are dealing with disease of one system, which is pointed to both by the *presenting symptom* and by the *associated symptoms* which have just been discussed.

However, in medicine there should constantly lurk at the back of one's mind the suspicion that one might be wrong; for symptoms can be misleading, and it is important to check that the system to which the evidence seems to point may not be the primary cause of trouble. For example, a patient who suffers from severe breathlessness at night may not be suffering from primary respiratory disease, but from a form of heart failure, in its turn secondary to high blood pressure. It would not be practicable to undertake in every patient a full inquiry into all the systems of the body, but it is a sensible practice to make a few general inquiries about other common symptoms which might point to disease of systems not directly suspected. This part of the history is called the *system review*. Examples of symptoms worth asking about are headache, stomach pains, cough, any problems with the bowels or urine, fits and faints, and so on. This type of questioning should perhaps be so phrased as to encourage the answer 'No'; otherwise a suggestible patient might leave with more troubles than when he arrived.

During the process of history-taking, there is a gradual transition from inquiries centred on the *immediate episode of illness* to inquiries concerned with the *patient* in general; and in a way the system review is a transition between the analysis of concurrent symptoms, and the concluding parts of the history, the *history of previous illnesses*, the *occupational and social history* and the *family history*. Throughout the whole process of history-taking a balance has to be kept between trying to discover the nature of the present illness, and forming a picture of the patient and his likely reactions to life in general, and illness in particular. In that context, the *past medical history* can give both specific and general information. As an example of specific information, a history of rheumatic fever in childhood (now fortunately rare) can point to possible disease of the valves of the heart. This part of the history may also give the general information that the patient is on the one hand prone to illness, on the other hand a generally healthy person.

In somewhat the same way, the occupational history can give both specific and general information. There are the specific hazards of particular occupations, including exposure to toxic substances such as lead or asbestos, or dangerous physical hazards in deep-sea fishing or mining. At one time, long term unemployment or on the other hand rapid transition from one job to another carried a presumption of instability, but sadly this now may give information on society rather than on the individual.

Akin to the occupational history in some ways is the social history, in which we try to discover something about the patient's environment, housing and general way of life, including his habits, with particular reference to tobacco, alcohol or other drugs of addiction. In taking the history on this matter, it is well to avoid any display of disapproval, both in the tone of voice and phrasing of the question, whatever one's personal feelings may be; otherwise, the patient will feel no compulsion to tell the truth.

The family history, except when it promises to be particularly relevant, as in some of the hereditary conditions mentioned in chapter 3, can really be confined to the age and cause of death of former relatives, and the ages and any notable illness of surviving ones. Some conditions, such as extreme obesity, can run in families; but this is not necessarily due to heredity, but possibly to family habits of what is termed, in an ambiguous phrase, 'good living'.

Recapitulating, the main divisions of the history are the eliciting and analysis of the present complaint or complaints; asking about associated symptoms; a review of the major physiological systems; a history of previous illnesses; and the occupational, social and family history. Clearly, these will vary from case to case in their relevance and importance; in straightforward issues, short cuts can legitimately be taken – a patient with a cut eyebrow might become impatient if you took a full history before stitching the cut. In the practice of a physician, however, it is vitally important to take a complete history in any case of difficulty; and students should also know how to do this. If you are seeing a patient for the first time, a careful history gives vital information both on the episode of illness and on the character of the patient; so that at the end of it you may have at your disposal the same kind of assessment as the general practitioner may already possess from his knowledge of the family background. It has also been my experience from time to time that a patient may, in the relatively alien atmosphere of a hospital outpatient clinic, tell things about himself or herself which they may not have divulged to a doctor who lives near them. If such confidences are to be made, they are just as likely, if not more likely, to come out during the physical examination as during the formal history-taking, when the patient may still not be at ease. So a listening ear must be maintained during the process of physical examination, to which we now turn.

PHYSICAL EXAMINATION

To an extent, this begins when the patient walks into the room, or as you approach his bed or chair. Anything unusual in the way he walks, or sits down, whether he lies flat in bed, or is sitting up on pillows, whether he is pale or high-coloured, the state of his breathing – all these things can have significance before the patient has said a word. And as he speaks you learn something of his composure and background; and perhaps more subtle clues, such as the husky voice of the patient with myxoedema (deficiency of thyroid hormone, in which patients become slow-witted, sluggish in their movements, and feel the cold abnormally, of which another piece of visible evidence may be their piling up of clothes on the bed, the so-called 'snug sign').

When it comes to the physical examination proper, this cannot be adequately made by undoing a button or two in the clothing and groping through it (irrespective of what physical examination contributes to the total picture, patients often judge their doctor by whether 'he gave me a proper examination'). Of course, a local condition of one limb may not call for a full physical examination; but any medical condition which requires a full history also calls for a proper physical examination, with the patient lying down and suitably undressed. Modesty should be preserved for all patients, and especially for older patients, whose standards are closer to those of *The Times* and the bathing machine than to those of the *Sun* and the nudist beach!

There are four established routines of physical examination – inspection, palpation, percussion and auscultation, usually carried out in that order.

Inspection

As I have indicated, inspection begins the moment the patient comes into view. When the doctor sees the parts of the skin which are generally covered by clothes, however, he can tell whether a high colour is simply the effect of exposure. Also, it is easier to see minor degrees of jaundice or other abnormal coloration of the skin in the parts not normally exposed to sunlight. Various skin rashes may become obvious on inspection, and also scratch marks, indicating skin irritation. Abnormal swellings or pulsations should be looked for, partly as a guide to subsequent palpation. In thin people, the heart beat is visible, and also the pulsation of superficial arteries and of veins in the neck when the patient is lying down. If venous pulsation persists in the neck when the patient sits up, this may be a pointer to failure of the circulation, or to obstruction of the large veins in the chest.

Besides looking at the skin surface, the nails, lips and tongue, and the inner side of the eyelids should be inspected. For example, the nails are brittle and even spoon-shaped in severe iron deficiency anaemia. The finger-tips may be swollen or 'clubbed' in some diseases of the lungs. Looking at the inner surface of the eyelids may give a clearer indication of anaemia than does the skin. The tongue can be smooth in some forms of anaemia, and raw-looking in patients with tropical sprue. The colour of the tongue can also be significant in assessing whether the blood is being fully oxygenated in the lungs. It was mentioned in chapter 3 that well-oxygenated haemoglobin is bright red, giving blood its normal colour. Reduced haemoglobin is darker in colour. In cold weather the fingers go blue, because the circulation in them is slow, but the tongue retains its bright colour, whereas in serious lung disease it too would show a blue tinge, the mark of what is called 'central cyanosis', to distinguish it from the 'peripheral cyanosis' due to relative stagnation of blood in a part of the body. Inspection should also include the movements of chest and abdomen accompanying breathing. Both sides of the chest should expand equally during inspiration, and also the abdomen, as the diaphragm moves down. If there is notable disease of one lung, that side of the chest may be relatively immobile, especially if there is pain, and this can be a valuable pointer to later parts of the examination. Rarely, the diaphragm may become paralysed as a result of nervous system disease, and then the abdomen does not expand during inspiration.

Palpation

Palpation simply means 'feeling with the hand', which should be warm and applied lightly and uniformly to the surface of the body, not used as a weapon of assault with fingers and nails. For the special case of feeling the radial pulse, or of confirming abnormal pulsation suggested on inspection, the finger-pulp is used; but otherwise the flat of the hand is used, bending the fingers as a whole when necessary. Palpation is especially of value in two circumstances – the analysis of abnormal swellings and examination of the abdomen. Although a sizeable swelling may be visible, smaller swellings, such as enlarged lymph glands, are usually discovered only by palpation. When a swelling is discovered, it has to be considered in various aspects – its size, whether it is tender or painless, hard or soft, fixed to skin or other tissues or freely mobile, and whether the skin over it is healthy or affected by it.

Swellings of organs inside the skull or the chest wall are obviously not accessible to palpation; but the soft front wall of the abdomen allows abnormal swellings to be palpated, given that the muscles of the abdominal wall are properly relaxed. In thin normal people, the lower edge of the liver and part of the kidneys may be felt, also the bladder if full of urine at the time. Abnormal swellings that may be felt in the abdomen include tumours of the stomach and bowels and enlargement of the liver, kidneys or spleen.

Percussion

Percussion denotes the technique in which the fingers of the left hand are placed on the patient's body, and tapped by the tips of the fingers of the right hand. If this is done over an air-containing cavity, the sound made is high-pitched, described as 'resonant'; if over a solid organ or a cavity filled with fluid, the note is lower-pitched, described as 'dull'. The technique was described by an eighteenth century Austrian physician named Leopold Auenbrugger, the son of an inn-keeper, who noticed that beer casks were resonant when empty, but gave a dull note on being struck when full. The note over the chest wall is normally resonant, because of the air-containing lung within; but if part of the lung becomes solid, as in pneumonia, or if there is fluid in the chest, the note becomes dull over the affected area. Again, if there is fluid within the abdomen, the note over it becomes dull. If the patient is turned on his side, the fluid may gravitate to the lower flank, so that the area over which the note is dull varies – a sign known as 'shifting dullness'.

Auscultation

This comes from the Latin word 'to listen', and that is just what it means, though the technique has progressed from a cambric handkerchief through the rolled paper and wooden cylinder of René-Théophile-Hyacinthe Laënnec (1781–1826) to the modern stethoscope, the caste-mark of the clinical medical student. Of course, Laënnec's great contribution was not only to hear but to think about what he heard, in relation to what was happening in the air passages of the chest; in that context, we can hear the air going in and out of the lungs, and also added sounds, both moist and dry. For example, in an attack of asthma, the bronchial passages are narrowed and impede the passage of air, especially on expiration, when the passages themselves are compressed; so the expiratory sound is prolonged and accompanied by a wheeze, known as a 'rhonchus'.

The other great area for auscultation is of course what was once described as 'sounding the heart'. There are two clear sounds in the normal heart cycle, one during contraction or 'systole', the other signalling the beginning of relaxation or 'diastole'. Disease of the heart valves can cause turbulence in the blood stream, giving rise to murmurs, and from the timing of these it is possible to tell whether there is narrowing of the valve, with obstruction to the onward flow of blood (stenosis of the valve); or whether the valve is leaky when it should be firmly closed, allowing backward flow of blood (incompetence of the valve). For each of the four heart valves, there are areas on the front of the chest where sounds emanating from that valve are best heard.

In addition to giving information on diseases of the heart and lungs, auscultation can tell us whether bowel sounds are increased (as may happen in obstruction of the bowel) or absent (as may happen in peritonitis). Something else we can hear is if there is an abnormal passage directly between an artery and vein in any part of the body; if so blood rushes through, causing a loud murmur.

Although these four standard techniques of physical examination have been described in succession, they are part of a continuous process of assessment, and can each contribute to the final judgement. For example, a very large spleen, say from chronic malaria, or a very large left kidney, say from multiple cysts, could form a visible swelling on the left side of the abdomen in a thin person. In distinguishing between these two possibilities, palpation could give some help, either by detecting the irregularity of a kidney containing numerous large cysts, or by feeling the notch which is often present on the front of the spleen (though it becomes easier to feel when other evidence has pointed to the spleen). Percussion can also contribute, because normally the spleen lies nearest the front of the body, the gas-containing (and therefore resonant) large bowel comes next and the kidney lies furthest back. Provided that the swelling is not so great as to derange this order, the percussion note should be dull over an enlarged spleen, and resonant over an enlarged kidney. Auscultation is of little help, except when, as can occur, the surface of the spleen is inflamed, and a friction rub could be heard over it; this would not happen with a cystic kidney.

There are of course important physical examinations other than the four basic techniques. Ordinary inspection can be extended to the retina of the eye by the ophthalmoscope, and to the outer ear and the ear drum by the auriscope, which are both in general use. For at least 50 years, it has been possible to pass rigid viewing instruments into the oesophagus, stomach, bronchial passages and lower bowel, although with considerable discomfort to the patient. This whole field has now been revolutionized however by fibre-optic endoscopy, which allows relatively comfortable inspection of virtually the entire alimentary tract. Palpation can also be extended to within the rectum and vagina.

Another important body of tests is used to explore the functioning of the nervous system. The cranial nerves are tested for smell, taste, hearing, vision and sensation of the skin areas and movement of the muscles which they supply. Similar sensory and motor testing is applied to other parts of the body, and a whole series of reflexes can be tested, of which the knee-jerk is the most familiar. The localization of lesions within the nervous system is one of the most intriguing tasks remaining to purely clinical methods of examination; the conclusions are now testable, not only by the surgeon or pathologist, but by increasingly precise methods of imaging – computerized axial tomography (CT) and nuclear magnetic resonance (NMR).

Again, I have emphasized the continuity between the information obtained with hand and eye, and that requiring instrumentation; but with endoscopy and the recent advances in imaging, we are clearly moving from examination into the area of investigation. Before discussing some of the techniques of investigation any further, I would like to make the general point, that after a careful history and physical examination, the time has come to pause and to make a provisional assessment of the clinical situation. This may be clear-cut, and it may be possible to proceed straight to explanation and advice to the patient, without burdening him with any investigations, or 'tests'. But this is not always so, and the next step may have to be formulating a plan of investigation and explaining to the patient why this is necessary, and what degree of delay and possibly discomfort it may involve. Depending on the nature of the investigations required, the patient should be told whether it can be done that day or at a further outpatient attendance, or even as an inpatient for a longer or shorter period.

INVESTIGATIONS

I shall consider here the types of investigation which can contribute to diagnosis, leaving until later any more general consideration of the impact of technology on medicine and of the place of investigations carried out as part of research, and not as part of individual diagnosis. In talking to patients, it is possibly better to speak of 'tests' rather than use the more specific term, 'special investigations'. This may also help us to remember that simple tests have their place in the scheme of things, as well as complicated procedures in the laboratory.

To take the simplest example of this, which may also serve as a bridge between physical examination and special investigation, it is useful to test the urine for the presence of protein and of sugar. In the old days this involved the minor hazard of boiling a urine sample in a test tube, but the same information can now be obtained by the use of dip-sticks impregnated with reagents which change colour in the presence of abnormal amounts of protein or sugar. For example, the substance tetrabromophenol is yellow on the strip, but turns green and then blue with increasing amounts of protein; and paper impregnated with glucose oxidase and orthotolidine turns blue in the presence of glucose. Similar tests are available to detect the presence of blood in the urine, and the degree of acidity. Inspection of the urine both by the naked eye and by simple microscopy can give information relevant to kidney disease and to urinary infection.

However, the majority of tests are now carried out in the investigative departments of clinical pathology, radiology, nuclear medicine and applied physiology. We have already met pathology in chapter 3, as the study of disease processes; but clinical pathology is more of an applied science, in that it is centred on the application of various laboratory techniques to the diagnosis of disease in a particular patient. The range of techniques is such that they cannot be encompassed in a single laboratory, but in divisions of clinical chemistry, haematology, clinical cytology and microbiology. We will take a brief look at each of these.

Clinical chemistry

This division is concerned with the application of chemical estimations to diagnosis. Chemical analysis can of course be carried out on solids, liquids or gases, but the great majority of the analyses carried out in the clinical chemistry laboratory are done on the fluid part of the blood, known as *plasma*. The sample is usually obtained by entering a vein of the arm with a needle, attached to a syringe, from which the blood sample is transferred to a tube containing a small amount of a potent anticoagulant (a substance which prevents blood from clotting). The sample is then spun in a centrifuge; the red and white cells sink to the bottom of the tube, and the straw-coloured fluid on top is carefully sucked off for analysis. Why are most tests done on plasma and not on whole blood, which would avoid the step of centrifuging the sample and separating off the plasma? The answer is that, apart from its high protein content, plasma is representative of the tissue fluid which bathes all the cells of the body. Changes in this fluid can affect the operation of all the cells in the body – for example, if there is too little glucose in the plasma, and thus in the tissue fluid, the patient will suffer from convulsions and coma; and any poisons will be detectable in the plasma, although their direct action is on the function of cells. This may seem a rather indirect way of approaching the essential problem, that of cellular function, and you may be wondering why we do not take advantage of the cells of the blood. There are large numbers of red cells available but they do not contain nuclei, and are unrepresentative of the ordinary cells in tissues. For a few purposes, where it is vital to obtain information on cells in the body, it is possible to take a sample of muscle for analysis, but this is rarely done because of the discomfort involved, and also because a muscle sample, unlike plasma, is not a uniform liquid, and this causes difficulties in sampling and in interpretation.

The range of substances that can be estimated in plasma is vast, but the most common estimations are of proteins (albumin, globulin and fibrinogen), electrolytes (sodium, potassium, calcium, chloride, phosphate and bicarbonate), urea and sugar. Automatic equipment enables many of these to be estimated on the same sample, and many other substances may also be tested for, on request. Since it is, perhaps fortunately, not practicable to do everything that could be done, the physician has a responsibility to decide which of the many tests available will actually contribute to the diagnosis. The choice may be obvious, starting from a clear-cut clinical suspicion of what is wrong; but in more complex problems there is value in discussing the choice of tests with an expert in clinical chemistry, and also the interpretation of the results.

For particular purposes, estimations can also be made on other body fluids, such as gastric juices, cerebrospinal fluid and urine. Tests on random samples of urine, apart from the simple tests for protein and sugar, are not of great value, because of the wide range of variation in urine volume, depending on whether the subject is thirsty, or sated with fluid; but for various purposes the total amount of a substance excreted in the urine in a fixed period of time, such as a day, can give useful information. For example, when the function of the kidneys is being investigated, comparison of the concentration of urea or creatinine in the plasma with the amount put out in the urine over a measured period can give quite precise information on the extent to which kidney function is impaired. A combination of tests can also be used to assess the chemical functions of the liver. In assessing the efficiency of the function of the lungs in respiration, some help can be obtained from estimating the amount of oxygen and carbon dioxide in the blood; but for a more thorough analysis, it is necessary to estimate the gas content of air entering and leaving the lungs, most notably that towards the end of expiration, which is representative of the air in the alveoli of the lungs. Chemically based tests are also available to study the absorption of nutrients from the bowel, and the secretion of digestive juices by the stomach and pancreas.

In addition to determining, singly or in combination, substances that are naturally present in the body, chemical testing is of value in screening for poisons, whether self-administered or the result of crime or accident. Foreign substances may also be administered as part of a test, the most familiar example being the glucose tolerance test, which may bring to light lesser degrees of impairment in dealing with glucose before full-scale diabetes has developed.

The broad indications I have given of the types of work that can be done in a department of clinical chemistry make it easy to understand why this is one of the most rapidly developing areas of medicine, which has benefited greatly from collaboration between doctors, science graduates and skilled technicians (now called medical laboratory scientific officers or MLSOs). The rapid expansion both in the complexity of tests available, and in the frequency with which they are called for, has made clinical chemistry a field in which automation of estimations, which I have already referred to, has been matched by mechanical methods of data processing and reporting of results. It is entirely feasible for a single sample of blood to pass through a multi-channel auto-analyser, the results from which are both centrally stored and printed out for the clinician, together with the locally determined normal range of the various constituents. A similar facility in data processing is now extending to laboratories of haematology and microbiology. The increase in the efficiency of clinical investigation brought about in this way has played a very important part in the development of modern practical medicine; but a plethora of results is not a substitute for critical thought, and it may be worth making a point which applies not only to clinical chemistry, but to special investigations in general.

Diagnosis, like politics, may be the art of the possible; but when we look at the bewildering array of what is possible in investigation, possibility has to be tempered by discretion. Diagnostic skill consists in reaching a correct diagnosis with the least possible number of tests, and not in ordering the widest range of tests possible to the certain discomfort of the patient and the possible confusion of the doctor himself. As we have seen, it is perfectly possible to do a dozen or more estimations on a single sample of blood from an apparently healthy person; indeed, this is a popular money-spinner under the evocative title of 'biochemical screening'. There are, however, both theoretical and practical objections to this procedure. The conventional 'normal ranges' for plasma constituents are generally such as to include 95 per cent of values found in a healthy population; there is therefore a one in twenty chance of a normal person producing an 'abnormal' result in a single test. When multiple substances are estimated, the chance of an 'abnormality' appearing in one of them becomes greater still. At the practical level, some 'abnormal' results can set off a wild-good chase which worries both doctor and patient. It is surely rather more sensible to find out from the patient what his concerns are, and to proceed from there along a diagnostic decision-tree.

Although the techniques used are different, similar

considerations of rapid expansion, with a consequent heightened responsibility for discrimination on the part of the clinician, apply to the other divisions of clinical pathology – haematology, clinical cytology and micro-biology. Again, as with clinical chemistry, I can only indicate in very general terms the types of activity in these departments.

Haematology

To begin with a general point, in many areas of medicine there is a fairly clear dividing line between doctors who work directly with patients and those who work in laboratories. The specialty of haematology is dependent on laboratory work to a much greater degree than most medical specialties, such as gastro-enterology, neurology or cardio-logy; the presence of a blood disorder may be suspected on clinical evidence, such as pallor or the discovery of enlarged lymph glands, but from there on confirmation and further progress depend very largely on laboratory studies. To the outsider at least, the distinction between a clinical haemato-logist and a laboratory haematologist is somewhat blurred, and anyone practising in blood diseases really needs to have a good grasp both of the clinical and the laboratory aspects.

The laboratory investigation of a blood disease begins with a blood count, with automatic methods of determining haemoglobin concentration chemically and enumerating the red and white cells of the blood in a mechanical counter. The haematologist also examines the blood cells directly on a film stained with dyes such as haematoxylin, which stains the nuclei of the white cells, and eosin, which stains the red cells. To put it very crudely, the two major abnormalities which may appear on a simple blood count are a deficiency of red cells and haemoglobin, or an excess of white cells. Unless there is some very obvious cause for anaemia, such as overt blood loss, the next step in either situation is likely to be examination of a small sample of bone-marrow, where blood cells are formed – if you find a defective product, take a look at the factory. The marrow sample may show a lack of activity, suggesting an 'aplastic' type of anaemia; or on the other hand, the marrow may be very active, yet clearly ineffective, as happens in pernicious anaemia, where the red cells cannot develop properly through lack of the substance cyanocobalamin (or 'vitamin B12' as it was called before its chemistry was deciphered). The essential defect in pernicious anaemia is a failure of absorption of cyanocobalamin, due to lack of a substance known as 'intrinsic factor' which is formed in the stomach, and which is deficient in pernicious anaemia. The failure of absorption can be tested for by giving a known dose of radioactive (labelled) cyanocobalamin and measuring the radioactivity in urine (a measure of what has been absorbed) and in stools (a measure of what has failed to be absorbed).

The conjunction of an active marrow and anaemia may also be due to increased destruction of red cells (haemolytic anaemia), and this can be tested for by extracting a small sample of blood from the patient, labelling the red cells with radioactive chromium, reinjecting and determining how long it takes these red cells to disappear, thus working out the life-span of red cells in that patient. The normal life-span is about 3 months, and this can be reduced to a third or less in haemolytic anaemia.

If the problem thrown up by the blood count is an increase in the white cells, or *leucocytes*, the next step is again to obtain a sample of bone-marrow, to help differentiate the various types of acute and chronic lymphocytic or myeloid leukaemia, whose treatment may vary.

A much less common condition than either anaemia or leukaemia is *agranulocytosis*, in which there is a great deficiency of the polymorphs (white cells with lobed nuclei). This may be due to drugs such as amidopyrine, which should now no longer be used. The condition is a dangerous one, since polymorphs constitute a part of the defences of the body against bacteria. It can be suspected clinically from the lack of resistance to infection, but can only be confirmed by blood count. The chances of recovery can be assessed to some extent by noting the degree of damage in a sample of bone-marrow.

Clinical cytology

Cytology, literally 'knowledge of cells', is generally limited to the information that can be obtained by microscopic examination of cells and tissues. The visible characteristics of the cells in the blood and bone-marrow form a part of the evidence on which haematologists reach a diagnosis. Examination of cells and tissues by staining methods and microscopy is useful in other contexts. The most familiar example of this is the examination of a small segment of the uterine cervix in women to detect pre-cancerous or cancerous changes in cells. Biopsy methods applied to other tissues such as the small bowel mucous membrane, kidney and liver have diagnostic value in the individual patient, as well as having added notably to our knowledge of the natural history of diseases of these organs. When a surgeon is not certain of the precise nature of a lump, say in the breast, he may remove a portion of this for immediate cytological examination of a frozen section of the tissue, which may be enough to say whether the lesion is simple or malignant. Yet another important application of cytology is in the detection of chromosome abnormalities in a fetus or child; in this way, Down's syndrome could be detected early in pregnancy, or the diagnosis confirmed soon after birth. It is possible to distinguish male cells from female cells by finding in the latter a small dense chromatin mass, representing an inactive X chromosome, and termed the Barr body after its Canadian discoverer. There are of course easier ways as a rule of distinguishing male and female children, but some conditions are known in which the appearances are misleading, and it may be important for further management to know the biological sex of the child. Biological sex as judged by cytology may be out of match with both the appearance of the individual and his or her psychological bent; here cytology offers precision in ascertaining one of these elements.

In the past few decades the scope of cytology has been considerably extended by two sets of advances; one of these has been a great increase of possible magnification, the other the elaboration of *histochemistry*, which means the elucidation of the chemical structure of cells and tissues by staining methods.

The magnification obtained with the high-powered lens of a good light microscope is of the order of 400, and this will show a good deal of cellular detail. But the electron microscope allows magnification of around 20,000, a fifty-fold increase, and this brings out details of the structure of cell membranes and of sub-cellular organelles which were previously inaccessible. For example, many forms of kidney disease are characterized by leakage of albumin through the membrane which separates plasma circulating in the capillaries of the glomerular tuft from the space outside them in which urine begins to be formed. Electron microscopy has shown up changes in the structure of the membrane in disease which were inaccessible to the light microscope.

The affinity of different cellular components for aniline dyes has been known and used for a long time, and a good deal of it relates to the acidity or alkalinity of the particular component. More recently, use has been made of the staining properties of the products of activity of the substances known as enzymes, which are biological catalysts, protein substances with the property of very greatly speeding up particular chemical reactions. One such enzyme is phosphatase, which can not only be estimated chemically in the plasma, but can also be detected in cells by appropriate histochemical techniques.

Another extension of histochemistry is *immunohistology*, in which tissue slices suspected of containing a particular substance with antigenic properties are bathed in fluid containing the appropriate antibody which has been combined with fluorescein. If the antigen is present, the antibody binds to it, and the fluorescein which is bound with it can be revealed by the use of a microscope with fluorescent light. This technique also shows the precise part of the cell or tissue in which the substance being investigated is located.

Microbiology

In moments of ease and carelessness we may speak of the 'conquest of infection', and this may even be a way of reflecting our relief at escaping from the time, only 50 years ago, when there was no direct and effective treatment for diseases such as pneumonia, tuberculosis, bacterial endocarditis and septicaemia, which caused many thousands of deaths each year. Nevertheless, the phrase is a dangerous one, if it is taken to mean that infections with bacteria and viruses have lost their importance. New bacteria, such as that which causes the form of pneumonia known as Legionnaire's disease, appear; and so do viruses which are new to the developed countries, derived either from simian hosts, like the virus of Marburg fever, or from tropical countries, like the virus of Lassa fever. To keep abreast of these new hazards, and others such as the virus which lies at the root of AIDS, we rely on the basic and applied science of microbiology.

The basic science is of cardinal importance in agriculture and industry as well as in medicine and new vistas have opened with the discovery that the genetic constitution of bacteria and viruses is so labile that it can be manipulated to constrain bacteria to produce useful materials such as interferon and insulin. The first hint of the lability of bacterial genetic material may have come from the observation that bacteria, originally sensitive, had at times the capacity to become resistant to antibiotics, and that this resistance could be transferred from one organism to another. In a comparatively short time, this capacity for transfer of genetically determined properties has been turned to practical use; but unfortunately the other side of the coin, the rapid development of resistance to antibiotics, remains with us.

I have mentioned these underlying complexities, not to be difficult, but to underline the continuing importance to practical medicine of the work done in departments of clinical microbiology. We certainly cannot always attain precision in the treatment of infections, and in a remote and urgent situation it may be justified to give a broad-spectrum antibiotic for the relief of an acute situation. But to do nothing else is sloppy medicine, if a microbiological service is within reach. A swab taken from the site of infection, or a sample of pus from an abcess, or of sputum or urine, should be sent for isolation of the infective organism. Bacteria are everywhere, and may well contaminate the specimen; so it must be taken and handled under sterile conditions.

Even with all precautions, there may already be a mixture of organisms in the original specimen, and the stage of *isolation* is important. One way of achieving this is to spread the specimen thinly over a solid disc of culture medium in a shallow round glass container, known as a Petri dish; separate colonies may appear, and can be picked off for characterization, either under a microscope after staining, or by their ability to ferment different sugars. Identifying the bacterium involved is not an academic exercise, but gives a clue to which of the many available antibiotics may be most appropriate. This choice should not be left as a hunch, but should be confirmed or refuted by finding whether the bacterium will wither or flourish in a culture medium containing the antibiotic. In practice, the steps of isolation and determining the sensitivity of a bacterium to antibiotics may be condensed by addition of selected antibiotics to the culture medium. Another way of isolating bacteria is to take advantage of their varying requirement for oxygen – some bacteria will only grow in the virtual absence of oxygen. There is also available a range of selective media, which encourage the growth of some bacteria and suppress that of others.

In all this, there may be a crude resemblance to micro-gardening, but to say that is not to denigrate the process, which is one of great skill. Dealing with viruses is even worse than dealing with bacteria, partly because they are both ultra-microscopic and ultra-filterable. They require quite different conditions for culture, and they are not visible by the ordinary microscope, although they can be made visible with the electron microscope. Also, they share with bacteria, and to a still greater degree, the property of variability of strains within the same species; this property is well illustrated by the influenza group of viruses and the rhinoviruses, which cause the all-too-common cold.

Although the isolation and characterization of bacteria and viruses is a large and important part of the work of a division of clinical microbiology, it is by no means the whole of it. In many cases it does not prove possible to isolate the organism causing the trouble, and the situation can then be clarified only by indirect evidence. Infections stimulate a response by the immune systems of the body, one component of which is the formation of antibodies to the antigens present on the infecting organism. If a suspension of the organism is exposed to the relevant antibody, the organisms are destroyed, and may either clump together or even break up. These phenomena, known respectively as *agglutination* and *lysis*, may be visible, either as clumps or a clearing of a turbid suspension. These tests provide another means of identifying a suspect organism, and they also, when done at intervals of time, give information on how the body is responding to the infection. The detection of antibodies is also useful in giving evidence of past infection, and in testing whether an immunization procedure has been effective. The group of tests of which agglutination tests are an example are commonly done in serum, the fluid obtained when blood is allowed to clot, and they are thus described as *serological* tests; the Wassermann reaction for detecting syphilis falls within this group.

Other investigative departments

I have given a fairly full summary of the type of activity carried on in the various divisions of clinical pathology, partly because they make up together the largest number of tests, and also because they carry out their work mainly on samples, so that you, as a patient perhaps, are less likely to have come into contact with them directly. By contrast, the remaining tests are usually carried out directly on the patient, the longest established and still the most important being the tests done in a conventional department of radiology. More recent tests, involving the techniques of physics, are carried out in departments of nuclear medicine and of electrophysiology, sometimes grouped together in a 'department of clinical measurement'.

Radiology

The chief property of X-rays which makes them of value in medicine is their ability to penetrate the tissues of the body. Use can be made of this both in diagnosis and treatment, but only the first of these is immediately relevant to us. It may be said in passing, however, that the use of X-rays in treatment depends on their ability to injure and even destroy cancer cells, which are more susceptible to damage from ionizing radiation than normal tissues are.

The diagnostic use of X-rays depends on the degree of 'radio-opacity' of the different tissues of the body. If all tissues offered the same resistance to the passage of X-rays, the photographic plate which constitutes 'the X-ray' would be uniformly affected, and the negative would show no contrast. However, the actual situation is that some tissues, like bone, are densely structured and also contain minerals which strongly resist the passage of X-rays, and are described as 'radio-opaque'; while others, such as air-containing lung, offer little resistance, and are 'radio-translucent'. Denser structures show up as white areas in the negative, while tissues such as the lungs appear dark. Radiologists generally use the negative in their interpretative work, and there is no great merit in preparing a positive print from the negative, which would involve an extra step. Plain X-rays can reveal fractures of the bones and show up 'foreign bodies', such as needles, shrapnel, or even glass, which generally contains enough mineral matter to resist the passage of X-rays, even though it is transparent to light. They can show swelling of the solid organs of the body, and also solid tumours surrounded by air-containing lung. They do not as a rule show tumours embedded in solid organs, unless the tumours are of a size to deform the outline of the organ.

The scope of diagnostic radiology was greatly extended

by the use of what are called 'contrast media'. These are substances of high radio-density, which can either be directly introduced into body cavities (for example, barium meals and barium enemas), or which are concentrated within a hollow organ when given by mouth or by vein (for example, gall-bladder X-rays or 'cholecystograms' and X-rays of the cavity within the kidney, 'pyelograms'). By such means ulcers of the stomach or duodenum show up as protrusions of the contrast medium beyond the normal outline, whereas a tumour would show up as an indentation, or 'filling defect'. Stones in the gall-bladder or kidney, if radio-opaque, may show up on a plain film; but if they are radio-translucent, they appear as 'filling defects' on a film taken after giving the appropriate contrast medium.

All these various techniques give information on *structure*, whether that be normal or abnormal, and the information constitutes an *image* of the structure in question. The scope of imaging has now been greatly extended by the techniques of computerized axial tomography (CT scanning) and nuclear magnetic resonance (NMR).★ CT scanning was first applied to the detection of structural changes in the brain, and was able to show up changes whose detection would previously have involved the use of contrast media, with considerable discomfort and some actual risk to the patient. Its use has now been extended to the rest of the body, but the precise indications for employing the technique are not yet fully established. The use of NMR gives still greater resolution of the image of brain tissue, such that the small scattered lesions of multiple sclerosis can be made visible.

All these techniques involve an external source of radiation, or in the case of NMR, an imposed magnetic field. Another approach, which falls within the developing field of *nuclear medicine*, is to use *radionuclides*, or radioactive isotopes, which generate radioactivity within the body which can then be detected either by the external use of instruments or by measurement of radioactivity in samples.

★ Commonly in America termed magnetic resonance imaging (MRI) in a rather transparent attempt to avoid the evocative word 'nuclear'.

In conventional radiology and its recent extensions of CT scanning and NMR, the emphasis is on refining the analysis of structures within the intact body. The techniques of nuclear medicine, while giving some rather crude information on structure, are more useful as investigators of the function of organs within the body. For example, the renogram obtained with a gamma camera following administration of radioactive iodine compounds will detect changes in blood flow to the kidneys, or the presence of obstruction to the flow of urine. Observations using radioactive iodine can indicate whether thyroid function is increased, decreased or within the normal range. The use of labelled red cells to detect abnormal breakdown has already been mentioned. I would not, however, want to exaggerate the distinction between structure and function, or the methods which are suited to assess them. The detection of activity in an unusual site can give important structural information. For example, the uptake of radioactive iodine is normally virtually confined to the thyroid gland; but if there is a tumour of the thyroid, with retained function, and if it has spread to distant parts of the body, usually the bones, radioactivity could be detected over a limb distant from the thyroid.

There are, of course, important physical measurements, including imaging with ultrasound, which do not involve either X-rays or isotopes. These range from the simple measurement of blood pressure, which forms part of the ordinary clinical examination, up to measurements of pressure in the different chambers of the heart, carried out by strain gauges attached to cardiac catheters. Electrical activity of bodily organs is recorded in the familiar electrocardiogram (ECG), vital in the diagnosis of 'heart attacks'; and in the electroencephalogram (brain) and electromyogram (muscles). The collection and display of such measurements is an important part of the function of an intensive care unit, the precise array of measurements obviously depending on the nature of the case. The panoply of measurement may be awesome, and we have to remember that measurement in itself is neither good nor bad, and it certainly does not equate with meaning. It is a useful part, certainly not the whole, of the diagnostic process.

So far in this chapter I have been outlining the types of information which can be helpful in making first of all a provisional diagnosis, on the basis of the history and physical examination, and in due course a definitive diagnosis, when the results of special investigations are available. At one extreme, the problem may be quite straightforward, and a definitive diagnosis can be reached even without subjecting the patient to any special tests. At the other extreme, it may not be possible to reach a definitive diagnosis, even when all the tests have been done. A fair number of acute episodes of illness, such as upper respiratory tract infections or gastro-intestinal upsets, clear up without a precise diagnosis having been made, and are perhaps loosely attributable to one or other of the many viruses which can cause short-lasting illnesses, described as 'self-limiting' in a phrase which is useful rather than strictly logical. On the other hand, the symptoms may persist, in which case the patient should be kept under observation at intervals, the length of interval depending on the nature of the case. When the symptoms are severe, and the diagnosis uncertain, a period of observation in hospital may be needed, until something happens to establish the diagnosis.

Now I want to take up the difficult but important theme of how doctors actually handle the information in making a diagnosis. I believe they do it in various ways, depending both on the type of problem they are facing, and to an extent on their own temperament. In the simplest case, where an obvious lesion follows a known cause, the situation speaks for itself. This applies when an injury follows an accident, or when one member of a family develops the same rash as another who has measles or chicken-pox. That is 'pattern recognition' at its most obvious, but a similar process plays a part in other, more complex situations. Both by study and by experience, the doctor builds up a series of pictures, patterns or stereotypes of a large number of disease states; this prepares him to recognize similar patterns when he encounters them in an actual patient. This process is seen at its most obvious in the recognition of disorders of the skin, and of the membranes lining those parts of the respiratory and alimentary tracts which are easily visible; but the term 'pattern' can more loosely be applied to characteristic conjunctions of symptoms and signs, which point to specific states of disease. To give only one example out of many, the combination of loss of weight, a hearty appetite, excitability and palpitation might suggest hyperthyroidism.

The contribution of pattern recognition to the diagnostic process is important, and may at times be dramatic, leading to 'diagnosis from the foot of the bed'. It is also at some risk of being fallible, and within limits accuracy is more important than speed in making a diagnosis. 'Within limits' should be emphasized, for suspending judgement until you are absolutely certain is a scientific luxury which may not always be within the reach of the busy clinician. But undue haste in accepting the temptation of rapid or so-called 'spot diagnosis' may be more dangerous for the patient than waiting for clearer evidence. This is a matter of judgement, and depends on the urgency of the clinical situation, and – to be frank – to some extent on the temperament or 'style' of the doctor concerned; and also on the degree of pressure put upon the doctor by patient or relatives.

The degree of probability conferred by the recognition of a familiar pattern can be very high, but it rarely amounts to certainty. Wherever possible, the probability should be increased by the use of specific confirmatory tests, whether as a basis for sound reassurance, or for the prescription of treatment. It would, for example, be wrong to recommend either medical or surgical treatment for hyperthyroidism without having carried out appropriate tests showing an excess of active thyroid hormones. This type of progression from an initial clinical suspicion through confirmatory tests to a high degree of probability sufficient to justify taking action is not uncommon; but it represents the easier part of medicine, and by no means the whole of it. All too often, both doctor and patient have to live with uncertainty, which stems from two main causes – the imperfection of our knowledge and the wide variation in both the severity of causal factors and individual responses to them.

The imperfection of our knowledge has more than one component. Our stereotypes of illness may be inaccurate because of false observations or false interpretations; the past history of medicine is riddled with examples, and it would be presumptuous to suppose that our present beliefs and concepts are totally correct. We must not take this too far – the building medical practice now inhabits has got in it many more verifiable bricks than those which made up the classic scheme, based on the four 'humours' of blood, phlegm, yellow and black bile. But no description of disease can ever be perfect; and even if it were, it would certainly be so complex as to be beyond the recall of any single individual. This is why discussion with colleagues, a willingness to look things up and even recourse to mechanically stored information are important in difficult cases.

The second cause of uncertainty is variation, both in the causes of disease and in individual responsiveness to them. Infective agents of disease alter in virulence, or become resistant to the agents used against them; and new poisons appear as new industrial processes are developed. New conditions appear, such as Legionnaire's disease and the acquired immune deficiency syndrome (AIDS) in the past decade. Individual response to what may seem to be the same agent is variable, as can be seen in the varying severity of disease in individual sufferers during an epidemic; and more dramatically in the high fatality of measles when introduced by accident into a community not previously exposed to that virus.

These matters are cause for a proper humility, but not for despair. It seems to me not entirely visionary to suppose that while the apparently intuitive processes of diagnosis will retain their value, there will also develop in really difficult clinical problems a greater readiness to be assisted by the techniques of formal decision-making, and by the greatly expanded memory contained in a computer-held data base.

For these various reasons, it is not always possible to 'put a name to the disease', however gratifying that might be to doctor and patient alike. This does not mean, however, that nothing useful can be done. It may still be worth while to try to answer three questions: 'What is causing this?'; 'Are there any structural changes present?'; and 'What is the effect on function?'.

Attempting to answer the first question means going back to the circumstances in which the trouble originated. I remember years ago seeing a patient with wrist-drop, which can be a manifestation of lead poisoning. His occupation of demolition-man seemed unrelated, until it turned out that in the course of demolishing railway stations in the Beeching era he was taking a blow-lamp to Victorian lead-containing paint.

The answer to the second question (structural change) has been made possible in an extended way by the newer techniques of imaging, which can supplement the information gained from physical examination.

The analysis of impaired function can be of practical importance, even if we cannot fathom the cause of the trouble, for it opens up the possibility of relieving symptoms, even if the underlying disease cannot be detected or cured. Half-way house though this may be, it is of great importance to the sufferer himself.

Because of its intuitive elements, and also because it is most often an exercise based on probabilities and not a matter of certainty, it is difficult to give a precise description of the diagnostic process; and indeed, the diagnostic process is different in detail in every case. To conclude this chapter, I would like to give an example of the diagnostic process as it might proceed in a hypothetical particular case of a relatively common condition. I hope this may bring out the interdependence of the various parts of the process, and also its 'trial-and-error' component.

A man of 55, employed as a railway porter, and with a wife and two children, has noticed that he becomes breathless on a degree of exertion, which he had been well accustomed to undertake without distress. He also notices that he tires easily, when working in his garden; but he is comfortable when sitting in a chair, standing about or lying in bed. He does not need to sleep propped up on pillows. His wife has told him that he looks pale. These symptoms have come on gradually, the first suspicion of them going back three months. This kind of story suggests the recent development of anaemia, and a glance at the man supports his wife's view that he is pale. Even a superficial knowledge of the natural history of common diseases tells the doctor that anaemia from iron-deficiency is not common in the middle-aged man, though common in women who lose iron during their menstrual periods, in the formation of babies and at the time of childbirth. Further, the most likely cause in men of this age is loss of blood, not from obvious haemorrhage, but quietly into the alimentary tract. Leading questions discover that the patient has never suffered from piles, that he has had a good appetite and has not lost weight, but that he has occasionally had some looseness of the bowels, and the motions have sometimes been rather dark in colour, though not tarry. These symptoms raise the clinical suspicion of anaemia, secondary to loss of blood from a tumour of the large bowel. Review of other systems, and of the past medical history, shed no further light on the present illness, and the family, occupational and social histories are equally not contributory. Physical examination, which must include careful rectal examination, both with the finger and visually through a proctoscope, to rule out haemorrhoids or a rectal source of bleeding, shows pallor of the skin, tongue and conjunctivae, but no other abnormality. Confirming or denying the suspicion that he has a tumour of the colon (bowel) will now depend on special investigations.

The patient is told that he probably has anaemia, and that the cause of this will have to be discovered. He can have a blood count there and then, but he will probably need some X-rays, for which he will need to wait for a few days. In the meantime, would he supply specimens of the stools (for which he is given cartons). His doctor will be written to when there is any news. The blood count confirms the presence of a low haemoglobin, and shows further that not only the total concentration of haemoglobin, but also the amount of haemoglobin in each red cell is low, and the red cells are smaller than normal. These are features of lack of iron, and support the likelihood of stealthy loss of blood. The source of this blood loss is pinned down to some extent by the finding of 'occult blood' by chemical testing of the stools (which are not bloodstained on simple inspection). This ratifies the decision to carry out a barium enema, which shows a 'filling defect' in the right half of the colon. (Barium naturally cannot enter the space already occupied by tumour; such a 'negative shadow' is known as a 'filling defect'.) At this stage, the patient should be advised to come into hospital, for possible endoscopy and for assessment for operation. Such is the possible course of events leading to diagnosis in one fairly straightforward and common clinical situation.

5

Management

The result of the array of processes which I have tried to describe in the last chapter can range from virtual certainty of diagnosis to complete bewilderment. It is important, before we even begin to consider what should be done by doctors for patients – and this is what we have decided to call 'management' – that we should clearly recognize that in some cases the clinical situation may seem crystal clear, whereas in others both doctor and patient, for a time at least, must live with uncertainty. This is not the kind of admission which a doctor is required to make from day to day, nor is it one which honour compels him to communicate to each one of his patients; but I do believe that in his heart of hearts he will be a better doctor if from time to time he admits it to himself – it will certainly save him from arrogance and dogmatism.

It is also important to consider which factors determine in the particular case the degree of certainty (or uncertainty) that may have been arrived at when the diagnostic processes have been completed. First and foremost among them we must surely place the *clinical situation*, by which I mean what is actually wrong with the patient, or in other words the nature of the illness itself. At one extreme we may have an acute illness with a characteristic easily recognizable pattern, preferably with a simple and direct means of cure, affecting a young man or woman with no apparent psychological hang-ups. At the other extreme, we may have a slowly developing condition of ill-health, with no very characteristic features and no obvious means of alleviation, affecting a confused elderly person. Guess which of these two situations affords the greater challenge. There is, of course, a whole array of intermediate situations, but the features of the clinical situation which I have tried to bring out as leading to greater ease of understanding, and hence greater clarity, are acute as opposed to chronic illness; an easily recognizable pattern; a strong hope of fairly early cure; a patient with youth on his side, and who can give a clear account of his illness; and that disposition of optimistic stoicism which leads doctors to speak of 'a good patient'.

As you may have noticed, I have not been able to outline the factors in the clinical situation which make for greater or lesser certainty in the mind of the doctor, without bringing in qualities that are really part of the patient's general make-up. What the doctor brings to the situation, in the way of skill and patience, is also important; and so is the interaction between doctor and patient, of which I shall have more to say in the next chapter on communication.

The emphasis I have given to the uncertainty that may remain when all the diagnostic processes have been completed could be regarded as an excuse, made in advance, for a limitation which this chapter on management is bound to share with its predecessor on diagnosis. It is quite impossible to describe in detail what might be the appropriate action in the whole wide range of situations in actual life; all that can be done is to indicate the general nature of the ways in which a doctor can influence the situation in the interests of his patient. It may also be important to say at this point, having just recognized that on a number of occasions any doctor will find himself baffled and uncertain, that he cannot make that his excuse for leaving the matter. He must still explore the relief of symptoms, even when the disease as a whole cannot be cured; and in appropriate cases he must not hesitate to seek the help of a colleague. This obligation is more clearly visible to a general practitioner, but a specialist should also be well aware of it.

The last general point I want to make is that 'diagnosis' and 'management' are not exclusive terms, even if we have to describe them separately. The sequence of history, examination and if necessary investigation should be the first step in helping the patient. Thus, the process of diagnosis should be the beginning of management.

There is, I believe, increasing awareness both among doctors and among patients, that those conditions that yield readily either to medication or to a surgical procedure, important though they are, are only a part of medicine. In many chronic disorders, the accent has to be on the relief of symptoms, and on attention to such matters as the patient's occupation, habits and general life-style; and there is also a much greater recognition of the importance of giving whatever relief may be possible in the later stages of incurable illness. Both to satisfy the legitimate expectations of well-informed patients, and to fulfil his own professional duty, the doctor must be prepared to consider, and if necessary to give advice on a patient's occupation, level of activity and diet, as well as on the more specific applications of medicines or the healing knife.

Occupation

With the exception of their family life, a patient's occupation, and indeed in these days whether they have one, may be the most important thing about them. Evidence accumulates that unemployment can bring physical deterioration as well as the more obvious psychological distress. Unfortunately, recognition of this particular problem does not bring any easy solution, and certainly not a medical one; though in the case of patients with particular handicps, the doctor can give some assistance at the margin by describing the effect of the disability in some detail on the appropriate form, thus making the patient eligible for inclusion in the quota of disabled persons which employers are expected to recruit. Equally, doctors cannot do away with the boredom and frustration inherent in many routine occupations, which may be the only alternative to unemployment. In happier days, or at least in days of full employment, I very occasionally advised someone to change an occupation which was clearly making them and their family unhappy, and hence more liable to illness. But this must now be a very rare option, in practical terms, when the alternative may be not a more suitable job, but no work at all.

At the other extreme, there is a widespread belief that ill-health can result from overwork, or from stress. This is not a matter about which it is easy to feel certain, but at the risk of prejudice, let me state my view that if people are doing their work well, they can do a great deal of it without suffering stress, or incurring illness. On the other hand, if either external conditions or limited personal capacity begin to affect performance, then anxiety may lead to psychological and even physical illness. A further possibility is that expressed dissatisfaction with a person's job may be a mere cloak for marital disharmony or infelicity. In each of these areas, a doctor must tread with utmost delicacy. It may be cowardice, but I have never felt very firm ground beneth my feet in advising people either to take things easy for their health's sake, or to break up or renew a personal relationship. Sometimes, advice of this nature is sought in order to fortify or justify a decision that has already been taken.

Apart from the particular hazards of specific occupations, the general effect of occupation as a possible cause of illness is rarely open to medical intervention. The situation is different, however, when a definite illness has led to a clear need for advice on future occupation; one such situation is epilepsy or diabetes in relation to driving private or public vehicles; another is the period of *convalescence after a heart attack*. The extreme dangers to be avoided in that particular situation are, on the one hand, to allow a level of activity which may precipitate a recurrence; or, on the other hand, to convert a previously active person into someone who is reluctant to stir hand or foot, and extremely miserable with it. There is also to be considered the effect of psychological stimuli, such as worry, anger and anxiety, on the circulation, which may be just as damaging in this particular context as physical overexertion. Probably no two doctors will ever give exactly the same advice, and certainly not to every patient; but my own general approach was to indicate to patients the two danger signals of chest pain and of uncomfortable breathlessness, both of which they were likely to have experienced in the initial heart attack; to advise thm to undertake any physical exertion short of bringing either of these on; and to undertake any mental work which they didn't mind doing.

Any advice on occupation or activity should remain within the bounds of realism. The majority of patients whom we now see would certainly not have the means to take the following advice on the climate suitable for a patient with chronic nephritis, given in a textbook of the 1930s:

In this country, Ventnor or anywhere on the South coast from Bournemouth westward is the most suitable climate that can be obtained. Egypt generally suits such patients particularly well. Madeira or California are also quite suitable. The wind and the more violent fluctuations of temperature on the Riviera render it much less advisable.

Unless they raise the matter themselves, patients may be a little surprised when doctors ask questions about their occupation, and even offer advice on it; on the other hand, in any acute illness, patients do expect advice on what level of activity is appropriate. Should they continue working, or stay at home? Should they remain indoors? Should they go to bed? The relevant factors in making these decisions include the possible infectivity of the illness; whether it is likely to be made worse by the changes of temperature met with during travel to work, or at work itself; the presence or absence of fever; and most important of all, the way the patient himself feels. There are a number of diseases, such as measles or chicken-pox, which are so liable to infect others that they are notifiable to the medical authorities, and patients should be isolated. People with colds and sore throats, sometimes called 'URTIs' (upper respiratory tract infections), are certainly infective, but are generally left to balance for themselves the conflicting claims of devotion to their work and the risk of sharing their infection. If an apparently innocent cold or sore throat becomes associated with any considerable fever, the patient should stay at home, or perhaps go to bed if he feels ill. However, advising a patient to go to bed should always be a considered decision; physically, it represents a constraint, and psychologically, the label of 'being ill'.

Until recently, and possibly even now, too many patients have been confined to bed, and kept there too long, at the risk of stiffened joints, clotted leg veins and, at worst, passage of clots from the veins to the lungs, causing the serious and possibly fatal condition of pulmonary embolism. If children are really ill, they will stay in bed; but when they are reluctant to stay in bed, it may be better, and certainly more practicable, to let them rest in a chair in a warm room. Studies have shown that mortality after heart attacks has not been increased by reduction of the recommended six-week period of bed-rest which was conventional 20 or 30 years ago, to a fortnight or less; and early discharge from hospital after childbirth is now usual. Of course, it is in the nature of pendulums to swing, and our consciousness of the dangers of bed-rest should not extend to hounding the truly ill from the comfort of the sheets. If a doctor is in doubt whether a patient should be in bed or not, he can get considerable help from an experienced nurse; and even the patient's wishes should not be neglected.

Life-style

As used in a medical context, this is not simply a matter of affluence, Bohemianism, permissive behaviour and so on; it is the totality of behaviour, which may have an influence on health. It therefore includes activity and exercise; dietary habits; consumption of tobacco, alcohol and other addictive materials; and sexual behaviour. These matters are even more important for populations and for society than they are for individuals, and their general aspects will be considered more fully in the third part of this book. There is, of course, no hard and fast distinction between what is good for prevention and what is needed for cure. Bad habits are not suddenly transformed to good habits by the mere onset of a disease which they may have caused. Of course, the rigour with which the patient should be advised to give them up has to be tempered by the clinical situation. For example, a smoker with chronic bronchitis should be strongly persuaded to give up smoking; but if the smoking-related disorder has taken the form of an inoperable cancer of the lung, it may be both kinder and more discreet not to press the desirability of stopping smoking – kinder, because not depriving the patient of whatever may be pleasurable in his habit; more discreet, as not opening the way to vain self-reproach or criticism by relatives. Of course, if the tumour can be resected with some hope of recovery, the situation becomes different again; it is on record that patients who have had a lobe of a lung removed for cancer, and who have continued smoking, have died some years later from a tumour in another part of the lung.

While an acute illness may provide the opportunity for advising a patient or his relatives on matters of life-style, it is in the case of chronic illness that these matters are more likely to be relevant in the management of the illness itself. For example, regulation of diet forms an important part of the management of diabetes, whether or not insulin is a necessary part of the treatment; and patients with alcohol-related damage to the liver should be persuaded towards total abstinence. There are also special diets for other conditions, such as the gluten-free diet for patients with steatorrhoea; low-protein diets for patients in the early stages of renal failure; low-salt diets for oedema, and so on. There is also the special case of patients who cannot take, or retain, food by mouth; it is possible to maintain nutrition for quite long periods by giving liquid food through a catheter passed into a central vein, a process described as 'parenteral nutrition'. The 'cocktail' so given contains carbohydrates, amino acids, fats, vitamins and minerals.

Specific dietary measures, of which these are only examples, are of high importance in particular situations; but they may be second in importance to the overall level of nutrition. In developed countries undernutrition is rare, and so are specific vitamin deficiencies. The commonest nutritional abnormality is that form of malnutrition known as obesity. This is prevalent in all social classes, the luxury food consumption of the gourmet being matched by the beer and carbohydrate of the gourmand. While it may not be the prime cause of any of them, obesity contributes to the severity of a number of diseases, as diverse as diabetes, hypertension, hernia, bronchitis, heart disease and arthritis. There are some risks in an all-out onslaught on obesity by regimes verging on starvation, and a more gradual approach is required. Samuel Johnson and many others have observed that if a man is fat, it is because he has eaten more than he needed to; but this truism does not account for the ease with which some patients lose weight, and the difficulty experienced by others on the same diet. (Differences in metabolism must modify the simple equation of obesity with 'overeating'.)

Without in any way lessening the importance of these general aspects of management, and also the mental aspects of management, I will devote the rest of this chapter mainly to the general scope, and also some of the problems, of treatment with medicines; and also give an indication of the available range of modern surgical treatment.

PRINCIPLES OF TREATMENT WITH MEDICINES

Medicines can be defined as substances given to patients in order to influence the course of a disease favourably. They do this in various ways, either by attacking a known causal agent directly (e.g. antibiotics); by supplying something which is deficient in the body for some reason (vitamin and hormone therapy); or by altering physiological function in such a way as to compensate for the effects of disease (e.g. antihistamines, diuretics). The concept can be usefully extended to include agents given to assist in diagnosis, to induce anaesthesia and to prevent illness rather than treat it. It is common knowledge, easily confirmed by a glance at the British National Formulary or any similar compilation, that the number of substances used as medicines is very large indeed. To some extent this is due to elegant variation, and even to complete duplication under different names; but sufficient complexity remains to justify two important branches of medical science – *basic pharmacology* and *clinical pharmacology*.

Basic pharmacology has its roots in organic chemistry and in physiology and biochemistry, and it deals with the physical and chemical properties of medicines, the way in which they are handled by the various physiological systems of the body and the ways in which medicines act on these same systems. Clinical pharmacology has its roots in basic pharmacology and in clinical medicine. It focuses on the handling and action of drugs in various diseases, with the various side-effects which they may produce and, very importantly, with the assessment of the efficiency of drugs in particular clinical conditions, often using the methodology of the 'controlled clinical trial'. The existence of these two important disciplines, and of doctors and scientists who specialize in them, does not in any way mean that doctors in general practice and in the various specialties can afford to neglect available information on medicines and their effects; but it is the particular province of the clinical pharmacologist both to add to our knowledge of the effects of medicines in disease states, and to assist in spreading such knowledge among clinical colleagues.

Basic pharmacology

There is a two-way transfer of information between physiology and pharmacology. On the one hand, increasing understanding of physiological and biochemical processes suggests new ways in which they can be influenced by drug★ action; to give a recent example, the tendency of damaged platelets to clump together and initiate clotting, with possible blockage of blood vessels, can be counteracted by

★ In this chapter, and indeed throughout except where particularly indicated, I am using 'drugs' as a shorter word for medicines in general and not in the limited sense of 'drugs of addiction' – heroin, cannabis and the like.

the substance prostacyclin, which was discovered through analysis by Vane and his colleagues of the part played by prostaglandins in the contribution of platelets to the coagulation process. This information has already found application in preventing clotting in artificial systems used for maintaining the circulation during open heart surgery. On the other hand, agents discovered and developed primarily for medical purposes can be used in the study of physiological function; for example, the antihistamine group of drugs counteract many of the effects of histamine, including severe headache, but do not affect the action of histamine in stimulating acid secretion by the stomach. It is thus possible to study the maximal secretory capacity of the stomach by giving an adequate dose of histamine, at the same time protecting the patient from headache by giving antihistamine. (This approach has now become unnecessary with the availability of the direct gastric stimulant penta-gastrin, and of synthetic histamine analogues which are free of side-effects.)

Of course, the interchange between physiology and pharmacology is not the only way in which medicines are discovered. The desire to treat diseases goes back far beyond the comparatively recent emergence of scientific medicine. There were enough agents available to provide the content of a pharmacopoeia published in Baghdad in 869 AD, at a time when Arabian medicine was in advance of that in the West. Medieval remedies were largely of plant origin, but the more disgusting were of animal origin, including live fish and frogs; some were very complex, like Venice treacle, with well over 50 ingredients. The number and complexity of the substances used, and the likely ineffectiveness of most of them, must have greatly handicapped any critical evaluation, although of course the innate intelligence and devotion of the physicians of the day were not responsible for the inadequacy of the means available to them. But, as Dr Johnson observed, where many people are shooting at a mark, some are likely to strike; and from the welter of unplanned and unconscious experiment, there would at rare intervals emerge a therapeutic discovery of lasting value. A notable example was the discovery by William Withering some 200 years ago that an extract of the purple foxglove was of value in patients with dropsy, an observation which opened the way to the use of digitalis and similar agents in the treatment of some forms of heart disease. To extract this important lesson from his learning of a secret remedy for dropsy containing more than 20 herbs, Withering had to have not only a prepared mind, which alone is favoured by chance, according to Pasteur, but also he had to be a skilled botanist, such that he could say with modesty, 'It was not very difficult for one conversant with these subjects to perceive that the active herb could be no other than the Foxglove'.

It is easy to see that the original herbal brew, with all its unnecessary complexity, might have been handed down from generation to generation, had it not come to the attention of Withering, or someone with comparable gifts. I suggest that the discovery of remedies on an empirical, or 'trial and error' basis, is a very chancy business, even though it may occasionally yield something of great value; and the current cultivation of traditional medical agents has to be regarded as a low-yield activity, compared with the planned search for agents on the basis of organic chemistry and physiology. To a great extent, crude extracts of plant or animal material have been replaced by pure chemicals, justifying the term 'chemotherapy' for much of modern therapeutics. The vision of applying specific chemical agents to specific targets, encapsulated in the phrase 'the magic bullet', was first clearly expressed by Paul Ehrlich (1854–1915). Realization of this vision in his own lifetime was practically limited to his own discovery of salvarsan for the treatment of syphilis; but the approach which he foresaw is now the basis of pharmaceutical industry and of specific therapy. It would clearly be entirely impracticable even to list the individual fruits of the pharmacological revolution; but its significance can really only be appreciated if I indicate at least the major categories of drugs which we owe almost entirely to this approach.

Medicines acting on the *alimentary system* include antacids, laxatives and anti-diarrhoeal agents, all of which are in fairly common use; and also pancreatic extracts, suppositories and enemas for more limited use. The antacids may act by simple neutralization of excessive gastric acidity, as with the alkaline salts or hydroxides of magnesium, aluminium, calcium or bismuth; but preparations of this type, although very widely used, are generally less effective than drugs like cimetidine, which suppress gastric secretion of acid by blocking it at source. In a diet adequate in fibre and free from harmful bacteria and viruses, it is likely that neither laxatives nor anti-diarrhoeal medicines would be needed; but in the real world they are much used.

Medicines acting on the *cardiovascular system* include digitalis, which in certain circumstances slows the heart beat and increases the force of the heart's action; anti-coagulants; drugs for relieving angina, such as trinitrin or amyl nitrite; and drugs for lowering blood pressure. Anti-hypertensive drugs act in various ways: some by lessening the amount of salt and water in the body (diuretics); some by slowing the heart and diminishing the force of its contraction, by blocking the cardiac receptors which control the force and rate of the heart beat; some by antagonizing the action of the blood pressure raising hormone renin; and some by decreasing the resistance of the arterioles, excessive contraction of which is one of the factors in hypertension.

Probably the commonest group of drugs acting on the *nervous system* are those for the relief of pain (analgesics), and the hypnotics and sedatives which help people to sleep, a group in which the more addictive barbiturates are being replaced by short-acting diazepam derivatives such as temazepam and diazepam, whose proprietary name 'Valium' is a household word, but fortunately not yet a household remedy. Other important groups of drugs in this area are anti-convulsants for the treatment of epilepsy and anti-depressant drugs.

Arthritis in its various forms has called forth a response from the pharmaceutical industry which might almost be described as exuberant, especially in relation to non-steroidal anti-inflammatory drugs (commonly and understandably abbreviated to NSAIDs). These include aspirin, indo-methacin and ibuprofen, but also a variety of analogues, which may have in common an inhibiting effect on the release of prostaglandins into the tissues. More specifically, the accumulation of urates within the body, which is the basis of gout, can be countered by administering the drug allopurinol, which inhibits the enzyme xanthine oxidase which is involved in the conversion of xanthine to uric acid.

Hormones, some of which can now be prepared by chemical synthesis, or even made by genetically programmed bacteria, are used in replacement therapy, when the body is deficient in them. Insulin and the thyroid hormones are the commonest to be used in this way; but adrenal hormones, pituitary hormones and hormones derived from the testes and ovaries are also used. In addition to replacement therapy, the steroid group of hormones are used, in the absence of any natural deficiency of them, for their pharmacological effects on the circulation and on inflamma-tory processes; they can be life-saving in the acute situation, such as shock or severe asthma, but their long term use in high dosage is attended by severe side-effects.

In the section on microbiology in chapter 4, I referred to the responsible use of *antibiotics,* an umbrella which includes agents for the treatment of acute bacterial infections, more chronic infections such as tuberculosis and infections with viruses. Other important categories of drugs which do not fall readily within the framework of physiological systems, are *anaesthetic agents,* drugs used in the *treatment of cancer,* such as the mustines and folic acid antagonists, drugs influencing the *immune response,* such as anti-allergic drugs (cromoglycate and the anti-histamines) and immunosuppres-sive agents, drugs acting on the *skin* and on the organs of the *special senses* and *contraceptives.*

I have found it difficult to reduce close on a hundred categories of medicines to something not too closely resembling a list; and the exercise tends to involve bringing in a variety of polysyllabic names, which seem to be the mark of 'official' names of drugs, in contrast to the often pithy proprietary names. There is no need for you to remember all these; hopefully you will retain a general impression that the basic pharmacologist has got a substantial area in which to exercise his skills. But apart from the number and complexity of medicines in themselves, there are also problems inherent in their administration and subsequent evaluation which are the province of clinical pharmacology.

Clinical pharmacology

As with other of the various 'subjects' or 'disciplines' into which medical knowledge is divided for convenience sake, there is not a rigid separation between 'basic' and 'clinical' pharmacology. They are indeed linked by two areas of knowledge described as 'pharmacokinetics' and 'pharmacodynamics', two somewhat off-putting terms which simply mean the distribution of drugs within the body and the way in which they affect their target organs.

Drugs are usually taken by mouth, but they can also be injected under the skin or into a vein, given into the rectum as suppositories, or applied locally in the treatment of skin diseases. Except in the case of local applications, drugs have to be absorbed, usually in the small bowel but sometimes even in the mouth and stomach, before they can reach their site of action. Drugs are obviously not inert substances, otherwise there would be no point in giving them; they are thus subject to chemical and physical processes within the body, which affect their distribution within the body and the concentration of the drug in various parts of the body. For example, some drugs are bound to protein, which affects their availability, and which also partly or wholly prevents loss of the drug in the urine; others are combined in the liver with organic chemical radicals such as glucuronate, which may make them inactive, or may make it easier to eliminate them from the body.

It is a matter of common observation, and also of some practical importance, that different individuals vary in their reaction to drugs; in some cases, this is explained by individual variation in the rapidity with which drugs are altered to an inactive form. For example, the drug isoniazid, used in the treatment of tuberculosis, is capable of combining with the acetyl radical (the same radical as occurs in the acetic acid of vinegar), a process known as acetylation, and this makes the drug inactive. In some people – 'slow acetylators' – this reaction proceeds slowly, in others more rapidly; this has the practical consequence that the 'rapid acetylators' need a larger dose of isoniazid than the 'slow acetylators' to produce the same effect. Like the great majority of biochemical reactions, acetylation is speeded up (catalysed) by an enzyme, in this case N-acetyl transferase, and this is genetically controlled, rapid acetylation being an autosomal dominant trait (see chapter 2).

Genetic factors are not the only ones which can affect individual susceptibility to drug action by modifying the rate of inactivation; an 'environmental' process with a similar end-result is exemplified by the phenomenon of 'enzyme induction' in the liver. Many drugs, including the barbiturates, digitalis and some anti-coagulants are inactivated by oxidases in the liver cells; when such drugs are given, this enzyme activity increases, so that more of the drug has to be given to achieve the same effect; moreover, this effect spreads over to other drugs which are similarly handled. A patient who is on barbiturate sleeping tablets needs a higher dose of an anti-coagulant; and conversely may suffer from bleeding if the barbiturate is discontinued – as indeed it should be. This group of enzymes may also be induced by the habitual use of alcohol, which may possibly decrease the effect of those drugs that are similarly handled. Although enzyme induction is due to an 'environmental' stimulus, there is also a hereditary component in the response, some people being more susceptible to enzyme induction than others.

The amount of a drug in the body at a given time will depend on a balance between the rate at which it is absorbed, and the rate at which it is either excreted from the body or converted into an inactive and thus irrelevant form, as a preliminary to excretion. In addition to the total amount of the drug, it may be important to know whether it is evenly

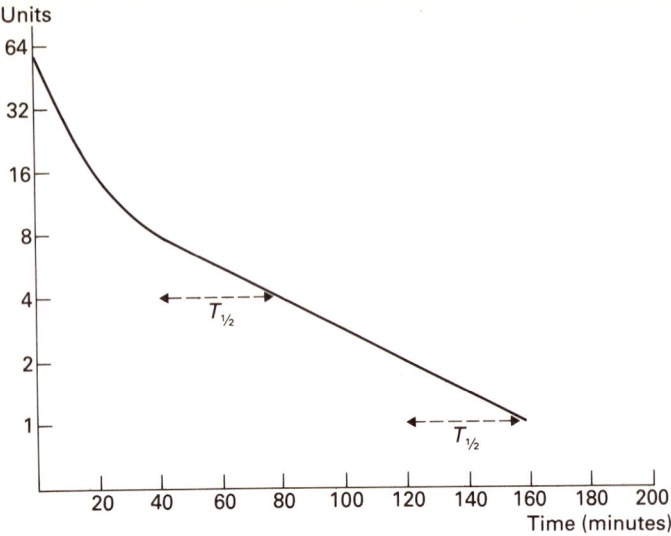

Figure 1 The concept of the 'half-life' (*T*½) of a drug. When a drug is given intravenously, its concentration in blood falls rapidly at first, as it becomes distributed through the whole or part of the body fluid. When equilibrium has been reached, the fall goes on more slowly, as the drug is metabolized or excreted. During the equilibrium phase, the time taken for the blood concentration to be halved can be derived from the slope of the blood concentration of the drug. This is the half-life of the drug. The concentration of the hypothetical drug, plotted logarithmically in arbitrary units, is shown on the ordinate (y axis), and time on the abscissa (x axis). Note that the time of 40 minutes taken for concentration to fall from 8 to 4 units is the same as from 4 to 2, or 2 to 1 units.

distributed throughout body fluid, or limited to a particular compartment of body fluid, such as the blood stream in the case of drugs which are strongly bound to protein. The broad lines on such matters can be predicted from what is known of the basic pharmacology of the particular drug in question; but because of the several possibilities of individual variation (of which only two examples have just been given), it is useful to have overall measures which can be fairly simply applied to particular drugs, and even to particular patients.

One approach in relation to the drug is to give a test dose of the drug and observe the time course of its disappearance from plasma; this is often expressed as a single figure, the 'half-life' of the drug, which is the time taken for the level to fall from a given value to half that value (figure 1). The drug is given by injection into a vein to cut out the influence of possible variation in absorption; and the measurements are taken after time has been allowed for the drug to reach equilibrium. What then remains is influenced both by removal from the body and by inactivation in the liver. The knowledge that the half-life of digoxin is about a day-and-a-half implies that a daily dose will lead to some accumulation, and must be adjusted accordingly; but determination of half-life would not be practicable in the individual patient. What is practicable is to determine the plasma level in that patient, and see that it falls within the known effective range, without trespassing into levels known to cause toxic effects, nor on the other hand falling below a useful level. By such means, it was discovered that different preparations of digitalis could vary in their 'bio-availability', i.e. the same apparent doses might produce different plasma levels, even in the same patient.

Pharmacokinetic factors of the type we have been discussing are probably more important than pharmaco-dynamic factors in determining individual susceptibility to drugs; but pharmacodynamic factors are also important, especially when several drugs are being given simultaneously. This can be advantageous, as when a thiazide diuretic (which tends to promote loss of potassium in the urine) is combined with an aldosterone antagonist (which tends to conserve potassium) – both of these promoting the desired loss of sodium in the urine. There are also, however, pharmaco-dynamically based harmful drug interactions, such as that between aspirin and warfarin, which impair different steps in the coagulation process, so that the combination may cause significant bleeding. This is only one example of a number of interactions between drugs which may cause harm. At the practical level, it is important to remember the possibility that a patient may already be under treatment for a longstanding illness; he should always be asked whether he is already on treatment from another doctor, before medication is decided on. This is particularly important in elderly patients, who may have acquired a number of medications during a long life, and may also forget to disclose them, or do so in a confused way. Careful questioning of patients and relatives is needed here, with the ultimate objective of simplifying the drug treatment as much as possible, to lessen any chance of confusion in taking the drugs.

In the last analysis, the effectiveness of a drug in a given patient for a given condition can only be determined by individual trial; but a part of the decision to treat rests on experience of the general properties of the drug, and of its effects on other patients. Sadly, the past history of medicine is strewn with remedies which appeared to do good, were believed to be effective, only to be discarded as experience grew. This has led to cynical pieces of advice, such as 'Use new remedies, while they are still working'. There is an element of truth underlying the cynicism; as is well known to advertisers, the suggestion of 'a new formula' rather illogically increases expectation, and so may contribute to what is called the 'placebo effect' – the subjective improvement which can occur when a completely inactive drug is given. The placebo effect is not, of course, limited to new remedies; symptoms can be improved by remedies new or old given in such a way that the patient expects them to help. There is nothing inherently wrong with the placebo effect, from the point of view of the individual patient; but it has the great danger that it may be interpreted as evidence that a drug is effective, when this is in fact not so. Recognition of this, and also recognition of the great variation in the reaction of individuals to sickness, has encouraged a technique of assessing new drugs known as the *randomized controlled trial*.

The principle of such a trial is simple and reasonable – one group of patients with a given disorder is given the drug under test, another group of similar patients is given an inert tablet, and the outcome of the two groups is compared. Because of the placebo effect, it is important that patients in the trial should not be aware of whether they are taking the supposedly active drug or the inert 'control' tablet; such an arrangement constitutes a 'single-blind' trial. However, if the doctor giving the drugs has a strong belief in the drug under test, he may communicate this, without meaning to do so, to the patient; so the trial can be made more objective if the doctor also is unaware whether the patient is in the test group or the control group – this is described as a 'double-blind' trial. The technique of the controlled trial can be applied to forms of treatment other than medicines, such as surgical operations, but then it is not usually possible to achieve unawareness.

The controlled trial can also be used to determine optimum dosage, once a drug has been shown to be effective. There is no doubt that the increased use of controlled trials, instituted after the last war by Bradford Hill and his colleagues, has put the testing of the efficacy of new drugs and procedures on much firmer ground, by allowing us to discount the placebo effect on the basis of what happens in the control group.

It is not, however, quite so easy to discount the effect of individual variation, both in the severity of the disease and in the patient's reaction to it. In theory, this variation is taken account of by the randomization part of the procedure, in which the allocation of patients to the 'test' and 'control' groups is done at random. This works reasonably well when the pooled patients are all relatively similar, the illness does not vary greatly in severity and there are not too many factors known to influence the outcome – conditions that have been largely met in many of the successful trials, such as those on the treatment of tuberculosis or bacterial endocarditis. Even if there are important factors with a significant influence on outcome, such as the presence or absence of pre-existing high blood pressure in patients with heart attacks, the problem can be overcome by selecting sub-groups with comparable levels of blood pressure. However, it is not possible to have large numbers of sub-groups, and at the same time to have adequate numbers of patients in each of them. When there are a number of significant variables, such as age, obesity and blood pressure in the case of heart attacks, controlled trials of anti-coagulant treatment have given conflicting results, probably due to the impossibility of ensuring complete uniformity between the 'test' and 'control' groups of patients. Another practical difficulty in the universal application of the controlled trial lies in the recruitment of suitable patients, when the disease is an uncommon one; no single centre may see enough patients to mount a proper trial. It is, of course, possible to organize multi-centre trials, but this compounds the difficulty of ensuring that the 'test' and 'control' groups are truly comparable.

I am therefore sceptical of the claim sometimes made that 'no new treatment should be brought into general use until it has been validated by a randomized controlled trial'. At one extreme, a new drug may be so efficacious that it would be unethical to mount a trial which included a control group, deprived of the treatment; for example, penicillin was soon shown to effect cure in bacterial endocarditis, which was previously uniformly fatal. It remained ethical, however, to test different dose-schedules and the duration of treatment with penicillin, using the techniques of the controlled trial. At the other extreme, a treatment may be making so little difference that its effect is swamped by variation between patients, in spite of attempted randomization, as in the example already given of the large number of trials of anti-coagulant treatment of patients with heart attacks, which have given no clear-cut answer.

Although I question the universal value of the controlled trial, I am in no doubt that there remain plenty of situations where such trials should be carried out; in addition to proving or disproving the overall efficacy of a drug, they can give important information on the balance of advantage between favourable effects and undesirable side-effects, and they may also contribute directly to our knowledge of the disease because of the careful observation which forms part of any well-designed trial.

These advantages seem to me fully to outweigh the ethical objections sometimes raised against controlled trials. These are twofold – that the patients, and also in double-blind trials the doctor, are being wilfully kept in ignorance; and that the patients may be harmed by failing to receive an effective remedy, should they fall in the 'control' group. The first of these objections carries a formal validity, and it must be countered by explanation to the patient before randomization, followed by his consent to take part in the trial. The second objection is partly offset by the general requirement that patients in both groups receive the best available treatment other than that which is under test; but more important, a trial should only be done if there is real uncertainty about the efficacy of the new treatment. When that condition is satisfied, the risk of failing to receive an effective drug can be set against the risk of receiving a new drug which may not be effective, and which may indeed have serious side-effects.

Patients, and indeed people in general, have a strong and proper desire to know whether drugs on offer to them are effective and safe; but the answers to these questions are not always straightforward. On *efficacy*, some drugs such as insulin, penicillin and cyanocobalamin are so effective in particular conditions that a small pilot study on a few patients reveals the fact. Short of this, a controlled trial is the most likely way to establish whether the drug is effective or not, provided that it confers a reasonable degree of advantage and is not marginal in effect, in which case the controlled trial, though the most sensitive method of study available, may still not give a clear-cut result. The question of *safety* poses different problems, and is indeed unanswerable, if *absolute* safety is what is demanded. Drugs that are to be used either in man or in animals undergo very extensive safety tests in the laboratory, including tests on pregnant animals, in the wake of the thalidomide tragedy. Although two or more species are used, the results cannot with complete certainty be applied to man; the drug is next given to volunteers, and if no obvious ill-effects appear, it becomes the subject of a pilot study in patients, and probably of a controlled trial – procedures which give further opportunity for ill-effects to appear, incuding those which may appear in patients with a particular disease, but not in normal volunteers. Should the drug prove effective, and show no serious side-effects at the trial stage, it may be released for general use. There are, however, side-effects that are very infrequent, so that they may not appear even when a few hundred people have been given the drug. Only when thousands of people have taken the drug may some effects appear, based on the susceptibility of rare individuals; and there may be further delay before the association between a drug and a rare side-effect is recognized, particularly if the side-effect is one such as jaundice, which may also occur spontaneously. This possibility underlines the importance of continued surveillance of new drugs even after they have reached the general market – 'post-marketing surveillance'.

The conduct of controlled trials and the safety of medicines are largely but not entirely in the hands of clinical pharmacologists and of pharmaceutical firms. But the individual medical practitioner also has the responsibility of being alert to unexpected effects of the medicines which he uses. Not all of these need be harmful, constituting side-effects: discoveries can also be made in this way, for example the important family of drugs known as diuretics has evolved through various stages from the observation that an anti-syphilitic mercurial provoked a flow of urine. There is also an ethical dimension to medication in general, and to controlled trials in particular, as has already been mentioned. It is important that trials should not only be well designed (for a badly designed trial is inherently unethical), but also that the ethical aspects should be sanctioned by a medical ethics committee, properly constituted and independent of those with a vested interest in the trial.

SURGERY

I approach this topic with the diffidence appropriate to a physician who has performed only one surgical operation in his whole life – a simple appendix removal done as a house surgeon 50 years ago. I must add that the operation itself was closely supervised by the surgeon in charge, as an 'assistant'; and that the patient was observed almost hourly during convalescence by the house surgeon himself. But even general practitioners and physicians have to retain some contact with the onward march of surgery, because the wise or nervous patient sometimes turns to them, with the simple, difficult question, 'Would you have the operation yourself, doctor?'. An honest answer calls for an assessment of two matters – the extent to which the patient requires surgical treatment and the likelihood of a successful outcome, given that the need has been established.

The *assessment of need* is generally, but certainly not always, easier in an acute situation; but it remains critically important, and once again, diagnosis is the essence of the matter. 'Sentence first – verdict afterwards', is no way to proceed, other than in the courts of Wonderland. Let me give you two actual examples. A patient with jaundice and upper abdominal discomfort may be suffering from acute hepatitis (inflammation of the liver), or from obstruction to the bile passages by a tumour or gall-stone; in the first situation, an operation would not help, and would indeed be harmful, whereas in the second it would be necessary, since removal of a gallstone would effect a 'cure', and even a tumour might be removable. Again, the sudden onset of acute abdominal pain might signify intestinal obstruction, or acute appendicitis, calling for urgent operation; but it might also be due to pancreatitis, which can recover without surgery, or even to the rare disease porphyria. The distinction to be made in these two situations calls for consideration of a number of different factors, such as the nature of the pain, its duration, exposure to drugs or infection, and so on. Interestingly, computerized analysis of these factors, known as 'indicants', can lead to a correct conclusion with much the same frequency as assessment by an experienced surgeon or physician. Such a system has been made available to more junior staff in Leeds for the diagnosis of 'the acute abdomen', and has worked well. Other diagnostic applications of computer technology are available, but are not yet in general use.

Most surgical operations are not carried out in emergency situations, and are known as 'elective operations', underlining that a *choice* is involved. Ultimately, this has to be made by the patient, in consultation with his relatives and assisted by advice from his family doctor or physician, and the surgeon who is to undertake the actual operation. Although the surgeon's hand is no longer forced by an emergency, the decision on the need for the operation is even more difficult, now that there is a clear option of not having it at all. An elective operation is done to cure a life-threatening condition at an early stage; to prevent the development of serious illness; or to relieve pain and suffering. Examples of operations in these three categories are, respectively, the removal of a tumour; the improvement of blood supply to the heart by coronary bypass surgery; and the replacement of a painful arthritic hip. The third situation is in some ways the easiest, for the presence of symptoms does incline the patient to believe that something should be done. The second example is not quite clear-cut, for coronary bypass may be done not only to improve the general outlook, but also to relieve anginal pain that does not respond to medical treatment. The assessment of need is somewhat different in the presence and in the absence of symptoms.

When symptoms are present, and particularly pain, it is usually possible to form some estimate of severity, though this may be shaded by the knowledge that some patients either do not feel pain very much, or treat it stoically; while others see in every twinge the approach of the grim reaper (doctors usually come in the second category!). Naturally, the patient will also want to know the likelihood of success in relieving the relevant symptoms. He is then in a position to make his choice between continuing discomfort and the risks of operation.

When pain and discomfort cannot be put in the scales, the decision becomes more difficult. Prediction of survival is much easier for the novelist than for the doctor; but the doctor still has to make an estimate of two possible survivals – that if *no* operation is done; and that if the operation *is* carried out. The second of these situations involves setting the risk of the operation itself against the added time which a successful operation would give. For a number of reasons both these estimates are imprecise. Information on likely survival in any given clinical situation is obviously based on the experience of groups, whereas the doctor has to advise a particular individual. The same consideration applies to the risks of an operation, and to the likely survival after it. However much the doctor stresses that his estimates are probabilities, and do not carry certainty, the patient wants to know what is going to happen to *him*.

If a general view has been reached that the patient 'needs' an operation, either for the relief of symptoms or to increase the chances of survival, the next question to be addressed is the likelihood of a successful outcome. Once again, the predominant factor in determining this will be, as so often in other contexts, the actual clinical situation. No matter how brave and hopeful the patient, no matter how skilled the surgeon, life will almost certainly be short for a patient whose tumour has spread throughout the body. There are some definite situations, such as head injury, where the outlook can be determined with considerable precision by relatively simple observation of the level of consciousness, the movements of the eyes and the response to painful stimuli. But in most situations, the outlook is either indefinable, because of the number of significant variables, or the necessary analysis has not yet been made. Perhaps the best the doctor can then do is to make an honest estimate of the chances, and then perhaps shade it with a tinge of optimism, both to patient and to relatives. For a patient facing operation, it is not necessary to dwell on the imprecision of much medical knowledge; but one need not carry optimism to the lengths of the surgeon in the old anecdote who assured his patient that he would be all right, since the survival rate of the operation was 1 in 20, and his last 19 patients had died.

Having discharged my duty as a physician by drawing attention to the inherently chancy nature of surgical operations (a property which they share with medical treatment), I can now pay a sincere tribute to the tremendous advances which have been made in all branches of surgery over the past 50 years. Of course, the great milestones are familiar – hip replacement, coronary bypass surgery, renal and cardiac transplantation, microsurgery allowing the replacement of severed limbs and the use of materials to replace diseased heart valves and blood vessels large and small. These things make the headlines; but just as important, and important to much larger numbers of people, have been the advances in the safety of operations in general. After all, the patient cares more for his own survival than for the brilliance of the operative technique. Several factors have contributed to this – advances in basic knowledge, increase in surgical skills and improved support for the patient before, during and after operation.

Surgery has benefited as greatly as has medicine from the general advances in medical knowledge, and particularly perhaps from the control of infection, both in the wound and in the body generally. It has also gained from increased knowledge of how the body and its systems and tissues work. At a more technical level, the study of materials, and of engineering principles, has made possible replacement of the hips, and in due course of other joints.

Surgeons are now both better and more consistently trained, and this is a matter in which the surgical Royal Colleges in this country have taken a lead. As Sir Alan Parks, the late President of the Royal College of Surgeons of England put it, the function of a College is 'the maintenance of surgical standards, in the interests of patients'. Similar objectives are being pursued in other countries, in broadly similar ways.

An epigram attributed to Lord Moynihan (1865–1936)

runs, 'We have made surgery safe for the patient; we must now make the patient safe for surgery'. This highly desirable process both precedes and follows what happens in the operating theatre itself. Preoperative assessment comprises a general medical examination of the patient, and also specific inquiries about drugs to which he may be sensitive. If he has been ill before operation, any obvious deficits in nutrition or in fluid balance should be corrected, and if the procedure is elective, it may even be better to postpone the operation for this purpose. Treatment for pre-existing conditions such as diabetes or hypertension has to be reviewed to take account of the restrictions necessary before surgery, and the effects of anaesthetic agents.

With modern anaesthesia, recovery from operations can be surprisingly rapid, unlike the stormy postoperative courses of the past. Nevertheless, there are quite profound changes in the chemistry of the body after any substantial operation, and also after accidental injury; these include a wastage of body protein and potassium, and a tendency to retain salt and water. This 'metabolic response to surgery', as it is called, may not be severe in its own right, but it makes patients vulnerable to postoperative failure of nutrition, or any abnormal fluid losses. Patients are also liable to clotting of vessels and shallow breathing after operation, justifying the brisk response of physiotherapists as soon as the patient begins to recover. A key role in preoperative and postoperative care lies with the anaesthetist, whose task extends far beyond the administration of anaesthetic agents. The help of physicians may also be needed in dealing with hepatic and renal complications. I should perhaps add that the great majority of operations are followed by an uneventful recovery, particularly if adequate steps are taken to relieve any postoperative pain.

Although my aim in this chapter has been to keep the focus on the management of individual illness, it has not been possible either to cover the field, or to avoid more general issues in such matters as the assessment of drug efficacy and safety. It is now time to turn from the issue of management to that of communication.

6

Communication

In this chapter I shall be dealing with communication between individuals, primarily between doctor and patient, but also between the various people who may share in the care of an episode of illness. The matter of more general communication with groups or with the public at large, either directly or through the media, falls more properly into the third part of this book, which deals with the health problems of populations rather than of individuals.

I made the point at the beginning of chapter 5 that 'diagnosis' and 'management' are not exclusive terms; and it now seems appropriate to emphasize that both these related activities depend to a considerable degree on effective communication, in the first instance directly between the patient and the doctor. Indeed, it would not have been possible to give any account of the process of history-taking without mentioning aspects related to communication, such as the importance of establishing mutual confidence and trust between patient and doctor, and of maintaining it by keeping the patient fully in the picture, and warning him of any possible discomfort or interference with his routine or occupation which may become necessary. When rapport has been firmly established, as early in the process of history-taking as possible, that process will provide further opportunities for strengthening rapport.

COMMUNICATION WITH PATIENTS

A good understanding should be the aim of both patient and doctor, as it is very much in the interest of both parties. Of the two, the patient perhaps needs it the more, yet at the same time he may be at a disadvantage in achieving it, because of the worry and discomfort of the illness which has brought him to the doctor. Because of this, the doctor has a responsibility even greater than that of the patient for doing his best to achieve the good relationship which will allow progress to be made. It would be unrealistic to expect that every meeting between a patient and a doctor should blossom into life-long friendship; but at the very least there is no excuse for enmity, and the responsibility for avoiding this lies primarily with the doctor, as being presumably the healthier party in the meeting. The doctor must not, for example, assume that the occasional querulous, petulant or even hostile remark, made in the stress of illness, is a reliable indicator of the patient's normal disposition. Of course, doctors themselves are not immune from the annoyances of life, and illness may visit those for whom the word 'patient' is something of a misnomer. Nevertheless, both should try to keep such failings under control in their professional relationship, to their mutual benefit.

Bad communications corrupt not only good manners, but also good medicine. If doctor and patient find that they simply cannot agree, the best solution for the patient may be to try again elsewhere. Such a course should only rarely be necessary, and if it is the initiative should lie with the patient, and not with the doctor. The doctor has perhaps a particular responsibility to overcome any barriers of race, language, or social class which may appear to lie between him and his patient. I believe that too much can be made of these differences, given that what is in question is a professional relationship, and not, for example, going off on an extended holiday together, or living on a desert island. If lawyers, teachers and social workers can overcome such differences, I do not see why doctors cannot, at the very least in those matters which are material to the doctor–patient relationship. I realize, of course, that my own experience as a hospital physician may have led me to underestimate the difficulty a family doctor may have in establishing the more continuing relationship implied in the concept of 'the personal doctor', commended by Sir Theodore Fox, editor of *The Lancet*.

I have laboured these general points because I believe them to be more fundamental to good communication than any particular points regarding the manner or content of communication. People vary greatly in their vocabulary and in their understanding, and although in general these two faculties are correlated, this is not necessarily so. For example, a limited vocabulary may indicate a lack of educational opportunity rather than any defect in intellect; and on the other hand, we can meet with expensively educated men and women whose developed vocabulary merely delays our recognition that we are dealing with a modern version of Mrs Bennet in *Pride and Prejudice* – 'a woman of mean understanding, little information and uncertain temper' (qualities, let me hastily emphasize, that are not sex-limited, or even sex-linked).

Perhaps partly as a hangover from the days when there was very little that a doctor could do to influence actual events, there was until quite recently something of a tradition among doctors that it was unwise to say very much even to the individual patient, let alone to the public at large. This tradition is now, in my view happily, dissolving and in Britain at least much of the credit for this should go to Professor Charles Fletcher, who introduced in 1958 the television series 'Your Life in their Hands'. The somewhat stormy reaction from part of the medical profession at that time, and the acceptance which now prevails that balanced presentation of medical issues in the media is a proper function of doctors, are matters for later consideration; but Fletcher was also responsible, in his Rock Carling lecture of 1973, for pointing to the importance of communication with the individual patient; to the lack of training of medical students on this aspect at that time; and for suggesting ways in which communication between doctor and patient could be improved.

This communication is a two-way transaction, or rather interaction, in which information is received from the patient, and also given to him by the doctor. The two processes generally take that order, but not so rigidly that they cannot overlap. For example, it may be helpful for the doctor, in the course of taking a history, to indicate the significance of a symptom which the patient has mentioned, and explain why this leads him to ask other particular questions. Transfer of information in either direction, for it to be effective, calls for attention to a number of general principles.

As I have already emphasized, good communication can only be achieved when a reasonable relationship has been established between doctor and patient; this calls for effort on both sides to bridge any gaps in knowledge and social background. Like any other skill, communication seems more difficult at first than it may do later on, and this underlines the importance both of thinking about it, being trained in it and, above all, practising it. But it must still never become mechanical, and the great variety of human nature should protect against that. To the extent that the doctor may become something of a professional communicator, I think this is a part of his art which is best concealed. A medical consultation is not a radio or television interview, and an excess of overt professionalism as a communicator by the doctor may defeat its purpose.

I hope I have indicated, in discussing diagnosis and management, that these matters are difficult, and likely to call for both knowledge and subtlety in reaching any conclusion. When a conclusion has been reached, however, and the time has come to tell the patient about it, simplicity must be the order of the day. The object of the consultation is to help the patient, not to magnify the skills of the doctor in the patient's eyes, except in so far as that will increase the patient's trust, itself an important part of therapy. Charles Fletcher put it better when he said, 'An elegant and witty communication may satisfy the communicator but leave the recipient uninformed and unmoved'. Simplicity and repetition become specially important when concrete advice is to be given, and anything complicated should preferably be written down, and given either to the patient at the time, or in the case of a hospital consultant sent to the family doctor, sometimes both, if there is likely to be delay in the family doctor getting the message.

It is well recognized that communication is not simply a matter of the words which are used, important though these may be; the way in which they are said, and also the way in which they are listened to, is important. There is little chance of the patient losing interest; but the doctor must both be interested, and look interested. Other non-verbal elements in communication include eye movements, posture and gesture, indeed the whole ambience. I learned the importance of setting the scene correctly the hard way some years ago, so long ago in fact that it was before there was dialysis available for patients in terminal kidney failure. I was explaining the very grim outlook to the relatives of such a patient, when I became aware that I had lost their attention, and they were no longer looking at me. Somewhat surprised, I noticed that they were looking at a book which had been sent me for review, the title of which was, *How to Learn Medicine*. I realized that they had drawn a conclusion which was reasonable, perhaps even correct, but was not appropriate or helpful at the time. Since then, I have cleared my desk of all books which could be misinterpreted in this way.

Of course, special circumstances may modify the application of the general principles I have been trying to describe, without impairing their essential validity. Rather than shouting at a deaf patient, to the discomfiture of anyone else in the room or even next door, it may be better to write things down. When there is a language problem, direct communication may have to give way to the second-best of an interpreter, who may be a relative or friend. Unfamiliarity, nervousness or anxiety may be mistaken for stupidity; but at the end of the road it has to be admitted that the concept of 'average intelligence' does have the implication that some will fall below that level – a consideration which, of course, is not limited to the patient. All these things call for patience, which usually means taking more time.

A very special problem arises when it becomes the doctor's sad duty to show his awareness that, so far as medical knowledge goes, the outlook suggests that death is approaching. Half a century ago the conventional teaching on this matter was based on two principles – that the uncertainty of medical knowledge justified a statement of outlook (prognosis) that was rather more optimistic than seemed actually to be the case; and that the relatives should always be told, but only exceptionally the patient himself. The first of these principles has survived rather better than the second. Despite so many advances medical knowledge is still imprecise, and remarkable recoveries can still take place, as well as remarkable deterioration; so I never feel the compulsion to destroy all hope, until the imminence of death declares itself by unmistakable signs.

The practice of 'telling relatives but not telling the patient' now comes under heavy criticism on ethical grounds. A simple argument runs that individuals are sacred in their own right and that this autonomy confers on them 'the right to know'; and who has a greater right to know than the patient himself? Those who obstruct this right must be both arrogant and paternalistic. Against such an argument, some doctors are still prepared to put forward a more utilitarian ethic, that the patient may be made miserable by forcing on him information which is certain to distress him. Against this, it is argued that the professed desire to spare the patient from unwelcome news is really an expression of the doctor's quite natural reluctance to give it. Moreover, should the patient detect this reluctance, it will only make his misery the greater.

It would be cowardly of me at this stage not to give my own view on this important matter. I am neither an absolute 'autonomist', nor a utilitarian, but I am what I suspect most doctors of being, a believer in, or at least a practitioner of, what is described as 'situation ethics'. This implies that there

145

are few if any absolute principles, and that the particular circumstances should be the most potent force in reaching a decision. This means in practice that one has to exercise particular judgement in each case on what has to be told, how much has to be told and how it is to be told.

The general trend over the years has been perhaps to tell patients more and relatives less, for it has become apparent that to impose secrecy on relatives is a form of distress, and that relatives may be even more prone to emotional damage than a patient whose faculties may already be clouded. It has also become more customary to respond positively to direct inquiry by the patient, even at the expense of inducing considerable depression, as surveys have shown may happen. In this difficult area, an important influence has been the growth of the hospice movement, which has brought two particular insights to the situation – that an open and caring environment can ease the approach of death, and that in a potentially painful illness such as some forms (but by no means all forms) of cancer, analgesics should be given to forestall pain, and often given by mouth.

There is of course no way actually to convert bad news into good, so at the conclusion of this section on doctor–patient communication it may be worth stressing that patients are as likely to over-estimate the gravity of any situation as they are to under-estimate it, so that doctors do sometimes have the pleasure of reassuring people. It may not always be as easy as it might seem to convince people that reassurances are valid; and to give good news convincingly may be as difficult as to decide what is to be done about bad news. The value of soundly based reassurance, which implies sufficient knowledge and experience to make it valid, is very obvious; but since its value cannot be quantified, it tends to be neglected by those who weigh the value of medicine in the balance of economics. Lawyers and actuaries can give working assessments of the value of a given life; but even they cannot express the relief of anxiety in pounds and pence.

COMMUNICATION WITH OTHER HEALTH PROFESSIONALS

Although direct communication between patient and doctor is central to individual medical care, it is likely that in all but the simplest episodes of illness help may be needed from other doctors, from nurses, from other health professionals and from social workers. When a patient is referred to hospital, he is entering a complex system, as is indicated in figure 2. Each of the possible transactions within such a system will achieve its aim only if the reason for the request is made clear. Some transactions, such as the request for an X-ray or laboratory examination, are initiated by completing standard forms, which have three basic components – a clear identification of the patient, a summary statement of the problem and a specified investigation to be done. For a routine type of request, this is sufficient; but for any special problem it is valuable to supplement the form by personal discussion between the referring clinician and the staff of the investigative department. When an approach is made to another department, not for a specific test, but for another clinical opinion from a specialist, the formal request made on a consultation form should also be supplemented by appropriate personal discussion.

Two types of communication between health professionals need special attention – that between doctors and nurses and that between the family doctor and the hospital consultant and his staff.

In the past, not every nurse attained the dominant position of Florence Nightingale; many nurses seemed content with an ancillary role, dutifully following to the letter the instructions given by the doctor. Times have now changed, for several reasons. Any young woman who embarks on training as a nurse must still have a vocation, just as in the past; but the feminist movement, which is one of the faces of justice, has seen to it that she will no longer accept a low rate of pay and meek subservience either to the superintendent of a nurses' home or to a doctor. At another level, specialization has come to nursing as well as to medicine. Now the

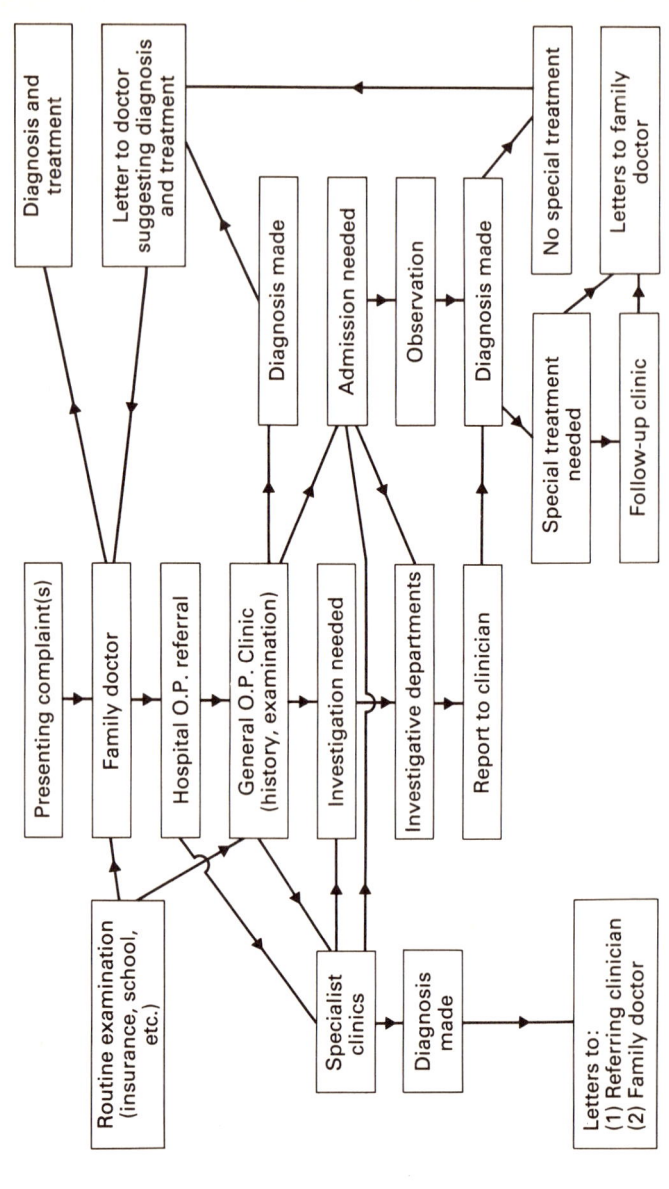

Figure 2 The possible channels of communication involved when
a patient attends his family doctor and is referred to hospital.
'Special treatment' is arbitrarily used to mean treatment which is
carried out in a hospital department, e.g. physiotherapy,
radiotherapy. When a patient is either admitted to hospital from the
general medical clinic, or is referred to a specialist clinic, it is the
duty of the doctor who has seen him to notify the family doctor,
who would otherwise think his patient had disappeared into a
limbo.

skilled nurse working in an operating theatre or intensive
care unit can be proud of skills which are different from, but
just as important as those of the doctors with whom she
may be working. University degrees in nursing are becoming more frequent and also a number of nurses have
graduated in sociology, which may have enabled them to
appreciate more formally that in relation to patients they
have a role which is complementary to that of the doctor,
and generally closer to the patient. Recognition of these
changes by doctors in general has not come quickly, even
though as individuals they must each surely have benefited
from the wisdom of ward sisters. Greater appreciation of the
nurse's role does not diminish that of the doctor, whereas
medical jealousy of the increased importance of nursing does
diminish the doctor himself, and this should be kept in mind
in communication between doctors and nurses.

There have also been some changes in the relationship
between general practitioners and hospital doctors, which
have a bearing on communication between members of
these two groups. Until the advent of the health service,
family doctors worked largely in isolation, and with little or
no secretarial help; while specialists were either full-time
employees of municipal hospitals, or attached to voluntary
hospitals, but dependent on private practice for a livelihood.
There was little contact between the two groups, except at
the individual level where a family doctor would tend to
refer patients to a particular physician or surgeon. Group
practices and a greater number of partnerships have lessened
the isolation of family doctors, and provided secretarial help;

and the development of postgraduate centres has given at least the opportunity for more frequent meetings between family and hospital doctors. The early training of family doctors now includes a substantial period in hospital, and many of them hold part-time appointments for hospital work. These changes have largely done away with pre-judices arising because the junior hospital doctors received scrappy notes from overworked doctors in the inner cities, but doctors in lusher practices dealt directly with consultants in nursing homes; while on the other hand, family doctors despised what were erroneously described as 'Poor Law hospitals'. Of course, not everything is sweetness and light even now. The 'please attend' type of referral note still exists, and conversely family doctors may apparently lose their patients into a hospital limbo, and be unable to recover them from a follow-up clinic. These residual problems depend for their ultimate solution on improved attitudes, but some attention to communication in either direction between family doctors and hospital doctors could help.

Family doctors cope by themselves and through members of the primary care team with the great majority of the problems which confront them. In the minority of episodes of illness which lead them to refer a patient to hospital, it is in their own and their patient's interest to specify the reason for doing so as clearly as possible. This does not as a rule mean giving an extended account of the patient's history, present and past; that is something for the physician to elicit for himself in his own way. Equally, it is only in rather straightforward cases where the problem is one of manage-ment rather than of diagnosis that the family doctor should give his own diagnosis; a 'second opinion' is likely to be more valuable if the 'first opinion' is not brought in to prejudice it. The important information for the consultant is the reason for referral and a note of any treatment which has already been given, with what success if any. These are matters which the patient may not know with sufficient accuracy. The treatment already given is particularly impor-tant, since the effective drugs now used may cause side-effects, and also it saves the embarrassment of the consultant suggesting a treatment which has already been tried and failed. In addition, the family doctor may be in a position to mention any relevant social or personal aspects which the patient himself might hesitate to bring out on a first visit to a new doctor in a hospital environment.

If the consultant, as I have just implied, has a right to be told why the patient has been referred to him, he himself also has important duties related to his reply to the referring doctor. At the very least, the family doctor is entitled to a prompt and courteous reply. The matter of courtesy is in the consultant's own hands, and it is wise to express thanks for the referral of what may seem to be 'a difficult problem in a difficult patient'. It is also worth keeping in mind that there are various ways, formal and informal, in which a patient might have sight of a letter sent about him to his family doctor. With regard to promptness of reply, the responsibility is shared between the consultant and his secretary. The consultant's life should be so organized that he has time to dictate letters either directly to a secretary, or on to a tape; preferably the letters should be dictated at the end of a clinic, when memory is fresh, and directly to a secretary, who can then ask for unusual medical terms to be spelled. In practice, however, letters may have to wait until an evening session with the tape-recorder. The essential item in the actual content of the reply is a consideration of the problem which led to the referral, together with detailed advice on how to handle it. Usually at least two letters are required, one to give a clinical view soon after the patient has been seen, and another to incorporate the results of any investigations.

It is specially important to send a 'holding letter' if the patient is admitted to hospital, giving the reason for admission and if possible an estimate of the length of stay. Otherwise, the family doctor may well wonder what has happened to his patient. At the end of a stay in hospital, a discharge summary should be sent to the doctor, saying what has happened; when there are secretarial shortages in hospital this may be delayed, undesirable though that may be. In such circumstances, the patient should be given from the ward a note to his doctor, setting out any medicine which may be needed. It is prudent to send a copy of this to the family doctor by post as letters send by hand may be mislaid in the confusion of returning home.

These all seem to me, and perhaps to the reader, to be matters of common sense, but since that is a rare quality, I have ventured to set them out, and no doubt others may come to mind. My final word of caution on communication between doctors is to make it as direct as possible, and not to accept without question secondhand reports of what another doctor has said. When I worked in a general medical clinic, I made it a point to ask patients what their doctors had told them about their illness, a measure of prudence to avoid flagrant contradiction of his view except when vitally necessary. On one occasion I was told that the family doctor had said, 'Your heart is breaking up, and going into your legs'. I found it hard to believe that these were the doctor's exact words, especially as the patient did not seem alarmed. When I went into the situation for myself, I found that small pieces of clot seemed to be breaking off and were being carried to the legs in the bloodstream – bad enough, but not as bad as if the heart itself were crumbling!

ASPECTS OF CONFIDENTIALITY

There are, of course, two sides to the coin of communication. The need to ensure that accurate information reaches those who need to know it is matched by the need to protect the confidentiality of information from those who do *not* need to know it, and worse still might even use it improperly. These are simple-sounding objectives, based on principles that are not difficult to state; but in real life circumstances arise which may make a breach of such principles the lesser of two evils. This final section of my account of communication must deal with the problems of data protection and subject access, as they relate to information on the health of individuals.

Legislation exists in many countries to protect the privacy of information, the relevant act in Britain being the Data

Protection Act, 1984. On the other hand, in many countries, such as the USA, there also exist provisions to provide access, under the general rubric of 'freedom of information'. The most general formula for reconciling these apparent opposites is one which provides access to those who legitimately require the information, and also to the person who is the subject of the information, but denies such access to others.

In relation to data on health, people with legitimate access can be taken to mean those who are sharing in the care of the patient, including social workers as well as health professionals. Excluded from access are those such as insurance agents, who might well have an interest in the personal health information of individuals but whose interests are not primarily those of the subject, who can however himself consent to disclosure should he so desire. The distinction may not be easy to make at the margin between those who need to know for purposes of care and those who do not. There is the further problem that records on patients may be seen by many people and what seems like harmless gossip may be transformed into a dangerous leak of information into the wrong hands. The obvious safeguard is a highly responsible attitude in all those who have custody of health records or access to them. Some of the relevant professions have disciplinary bodies, such as the General Medical Council, which can punish breaches of confidentiality. In the case of other employees this matter should be covered by a confidentiality clause in their contract of service. It also seems inevitable that data protection measures, which are at present limited to mechanically held and processed information, should ultimately be extended to manual records. This will considerably increase the number of people who will have responsibility both for the maintenance and confidentiality of records.

The principle of denying information on the present or past health of a patient to those not involved in the care of that patient (except with the consent of the patient) is in general sound, but there must also be exceptions to it, the prevention of terrorism or other serious crime being an obvious example in the lay field. The use of information for epidemiological research is more relevant to medicine, but it does raise a problem. For studies involving thousands of people, such as on the relation between smoking and heart disease or cancer, it would obviously be impracticable to obtain the informed consent of each of the subjects of the study, the difficulty reaching its height when the source of information is a death certificate. Hitherto, safeguards against the improper use of such information have rested on the integrity of the research workers involved, together with scrutiny of the proposed research by an ethical committee; there is also no question of revealing the identity of the subjects of the data in any published material. I think the present state of affairs is satisfactory, and that the consent of the data subjects to the unattributable use of information on them can be implied from their having sought access to health care; but there is another view, that consent should always be directly obtained, whatever the difficulties.

Other problems surround the matter of what is termed 'subject access', by which is meant the right of a patient to see his record. Although it may seem like natural justice, this is not a right that has been freely accorded in the past, the argument being that such access might cause distress to a patient who discovers that he is suffering from a serious disease, unsuspected by him; or that he might unearth a note that he was less than perfect, or perhaps even unreliable, in recounting his history. To take the second of these first, comment on the patient's virtues or vices in giving their story can be useful either to the note-taker when the patient is seen again after an interval, or when some other doctor sees him, as is often the case in a hospital clinic, however undesirable exposure to a succession of doctors may be. The matter of distress through learning about an unsuspected illness is both more common and more important, and perhaps also more difficult to deal with. I am old-fashioned enough to believe that normally the doctor should give the patient an explanation, using the record but not displaying it. If the patient is not then satisfied, he should be encouraged to seek a further medical opinion, and thus receive an independent interpretation of the record, which will be shown to the second doctor. Should the patient still be unhappy, however, and even suspect that the two doctors are in collusion, he should in the last resort have a right of access, possibly through the courts. But this is a less than perfect solution, because the bare record may be of little value without interpretation. The possible discovery of unpalatable information is perhaps at this stage less serious, since anyone who has had the persistence to go through these stages of discovery may not be too readily upset. In the real world, however, it is rare for a patient to seek access to his record, and when he does it suggests that the doctor–patient relationship is already under strain.

PART III

The Application of Medical Knowledge to Populations

In Part II I considered the application of medical knowledge and skills to the needs of individuals. Medical knowledge is also relevant to some of the needs of people not considered individually, but aggregated into populations. The application of medical knowledge to the needs of populations, however, calls for skills that are in some ways different from those required to make the benefits of medical knowledge available to individuals. There are also significant differences in the underlying scientific disciplines on which the greatest emphasis has to be laid. Put summarily, the practice of individual or personal medicine, to the extent that it is scientific, is based on anatomy, physiology, biochemistry and pathology; the application of medical knowledge to populations requires disciplines such as epidemiology, sociology and economics. The distinction between individual and population medicine, in other words, lies not so much in the nature of medical knowledge, which should be common to both, but in the skills needed to select from the corpus of medical knowledge what is most relevant, and to apply it most effectively.

We mostly know what we mean by 'individuals', and we have a sense that we can generally relate to them on a personal level; but out ideas of what constitutes a 'population', and of how we relate to that, are distinctly more remote and abstract. In a very general sense, any group of people may constitute 'a population'; but the sort of random aggregations you might meet on a railway station or at a party are not populations that would be appropriate for scientific study, since they would probably lack important common characteristics (other than simply being 'human'), and they would also sooner or later disperse. In order to be worthy of study, populations should be 'defined' in some way, otherwise we are working with shifting sand.

There are various possible criteria for defining a population – geographical, like the population of a nation or a parish; the existence of a register, such as that of the patients in a practice; or by some characteristic shared by all members of the study population, such as occupation, environmental exposure and so on. The perfect 'defined population' is perhaps more an abstraction than a reality, because of movement of individuals into and out of it, and because the criterion or criteria chosen to define it do not exclude differences within it which may be very relevant. A further difficulty is that even if a population has been defined in a reasonably satisfactory way, it may still not be practicable to study each member of it, so that only a sample of the entire population can be used. The most difficult and even dangerous part of statistics may lie in the definition of a population and in the selection of a representative sample from it. Statistics is relevant to my theme, as being the scientific basis of epidemiology; but I am no expert, and I would recommend study of the companion volume on statistics in this series by Gavin Kennedy, which draws many examples from medical studies, and also recognizes the importance of defined populations and of samples in the chapter entitled 'By your samples be judged'.

In relation to individual medicine, we have already drawn heavily on information obtained from the study of one type of population, those adjudged to have a particular disease. Useful as they are, populations so defined are blurred at the margins, because as was emphasized in chapter 3, diseases are not absolute entities, so that distinctions made on that basis are imperfect – which does not of course deprive them of all practical value, in a world largely made up of imperfections.

As we pass from the individual to the population, and to

considerations of health care rather than of personal medicine, it is worth pointing out that for the majority of diseases the sample seen by doctors is likely to be only a selected part of a larger population. This is less true for serious and easily identified diseases such as major infections or tumours; but even so the patients are likely to be treated in different places, and special registers would be needed to establish a comprehensive picture. Moreover, for so-called 'minor disorders' the difficulties are much greater. Most illnesses, or deviations from health, are looked after by the patient himself, or by relatives and non-medical agencies in the community, such as the local pharmacist. The average number of attendances by patients in family practice is around two a year; but this average conceals wide variations, from the patient who does not see his doctor from one year to another, to the patient who visits the surgery once a week or oftener. Of course a still smaller proportion of patients are admitted to hospital in the course of a year.

These well-recognized facts have encouraged a movement to diminish the place of doctors in health care, giving rise to such statements as, 'The doctor need attend only those 2–3 per cent of illnesses which lie beyond the capacity of an informed people and their health workers'. Not surprisingly perhaps, I have suspicions about the elevation of a system based on 'bare-foot doctors' in developing countries into a model for advanced countries. It is not always wise to convert what may be a necessity in one situation into a virtue in another. More practically, it may take more than 'an informed people and their health workers' to decide which *are* the '2–3 per cent of illnesses' which actually need medical attention. There is also a numerical discrepancy between '2–3 per cent of illnesses needing a doctor' and 'two visits per year' – if both were correct, we would each of us have an average of 60–100 illnesses a year! Of the two apparently conflicting estimates, it is the 'two visits a year' which is based on actual assessment, and indeed most people have only one or two illnesses a year, if that.

In this introduction I have only touched on two of the major themes of this third section, the study of health and disease in populations and the provision of health care. These are not matters in which doctors have any monopoly, and doctors cannot deal with them unaided; but I do maintain that there is an important medical contribution to be made in these areas, both by drawing on medical knowledge and through the activities of individual doctors.

7

The Public Health

Awareness of environmental influences on health is not new; for example, one of the writings which has come down to us as part of the Hippocratic corpus is entitled 'Airs, Waters, Places', and deals with the influence on health of climate, water supply and similar factors. The author contrasts the physical characteristics and health experience of Egyptians and Libyans on the one hand, with the Scythians of South Russia on the other, to quote the two extremes. However, the response to the ambiguous gifts of nature was then almost entirely an individual matter, be it by loose clothing and shade against the heat, or by fires and snug dwellings against the cold. In dealing with pestilence there was of course no knowledge of micro-organisms, and consequently only limited awareness of methods of spread. The intensity of quarantine, as in the case of leprosy, was determined at least as much by the severity of the disease as by its infectivity. The importance of a clean water supply, and the risks of a stagnant source of water were recognized by the Hippocratic writer; and the pax Romana brought to cities, and even to isolated villas, the benefits of a good water supply, for bathing as well as for drinking, and of sewage disposal. But much of the world, then as now, must have been lacking in such amenities; and after the fall of Rome it was to be many centuries before the same level of sanitary hygiene would once again be obtained, even in civilized countries.

The widespread recognition of a corporate, as well as an

individual, responsibility for health came only in the nineteenth century, in the wake of the industrial revolution. There had, of course, been men of vision before that time, such as Bernardo Ramazzini (1633–1714) in Italy and Charles Thackrah (1795–1833) in Leeds (who escapes inclusion in the Dictionary of National Biography), who recognized that society had a responsibility for improving conditions at work; and the adverse effects of industrial life and urbanization on health were recognized by Thomas Percival (1740–1804), a general practitioner in Manchester, who also wrote a treatise on medical ethics. The massive shift of people from the country to the rapidly growing towns and cities during the industrial revolution both manifested the need, and created the opportunity, for establishing an organized system of water supply, sewage disposal and other public health measures.

HEALTH REFORM IN THE NINETEENTH CENTURY

Just as anthropologists in seeking to reconstruct the conditions of life in primitive ages are helped by observation of primitive cultures today, so the masses of people living still in undeveloped countries may represent some kind of model of what conditions were like in Europe and the USA before industry, as it were, 'set in'. The marks of a primitive population, whether historical or contemporary, in terms of employment are a high proportion of the workforce engaged in agriculture, and within that workforce a high proportion of women at work on the land; and in terms of health, a high perinatal and infant mortality, and deaths at all ages coming mainly from infections, respiratory and alimentary disease. In an industrial economy, most people are engaged in manufacture, construction and commerce, and the proportion of women in the workforce is smaller, say a third rather than a half. In terms of health, mortality in the first year of life is much lower, and deaths in the population at large are due not to infection, but to the so-called degenerative diseases, or diseases of ageing, such as tumours, heart disease and strokes. In different countries, and even in different parts of the same country, there would be many differences in detail in the transition from a small scattered population, mainly engaged in food production, to a larger and largely urbanized population mainly engaged in manufacture.

In Britain the population increase had begun as early as 1700, thus preceding any large scale industrialization; and this was permitted by improved agricultural methods, and a higher standard of living from the development of overseas trade. While the general rate of mortality was declining, the rapid growth of industry when it came produced pockets of high mortality in the new slum areas. There was of course tension between the *laissez-faire* industrialists who would stress the general increase in prosperity, and those who would be more conscious of the evils of child labour, bad housing and inadequate wages. The former group maintained that 'suffering and evil are nature's admonitions; they cannot be got rid of', but the humanitarians were able to show that the prophecy of national ruin, made in opposition to each measure of reform, remained persistently unfulfilled.

Consideration of the reforms made in the nineteenth century which have allowed our country to maintain a greatly increased population in reasonable health is not just an academic historical exercise; it remains relevant in many ways. Two examples would be the persistence of social inequalities in health and the preponderance of 'social' over strictly 'medical' factors in raising the general standard of health.

True, it would now be difficult to repeat Lord Shaftesbury's discovery, recounted by Trevelyan, of 'a room with a family in each of its four corners and a room with a cesspool below its boarded floor'. Nevertheless, tangible health disadvantage persists to a very notable extent in the poorer sections of a nation. To give a specific example, the mortality in unskilled manual workers and their families in Britain in 1971–72 was between two and four times greater than that of professional families, the disparity being greatest in the first year of life.

As already mentioned, the decline in mortality had begun before there was widespread industrialization; this being so, it preceded by an even longer period anything which could be termed effective therapeutics, in terms of outcome on any large scale. Lister's introduction of antiseptic surgery did not take place until 1866; and really effective medical intervention in a common disease had to wait until the discovery of insulin in 1922. These events were of the highest importance, both in themselves and in the promise they gave of further effective intervention. They saved lives, but against the backdrop of the great killing diseases, the actual number of lives saved was comparatively small. Improved nutrition, better housing, good water supply and sanitation, and more humane and safer conditions of employment, these must have been the factors of most importance in effecting the improvement which undoubtedly took place.

Ernest Chadwick (1800–90), one of the most pertinacious of the reformers, was well aware of the need to challenge the obvious dangers to health on a broad front. His 1842 survey on 'The Sanitary Condition of the Labouring Population of Great Britain' brought together evidence of poor housing, overcrowding and lack of sanitation. Chadwick was also active in reform of the Poor Law. Like many people who get things done, he had a high zeal to tact ratio, and succeeded in antagonizing doctors, engineers, vestrymen and burial boards. His persistence, together with recurrent outbreaks of cholera, got the first Public Health Act on to the statute book in 1848, a year before John Snow's careful demonstration that cholera was a water-borne disease, and 35 years before Koch's discovery of the causative organism, *Vibrio cholerae*. This is not an isolated example of the possibility of effective empirical action preceding the establishment of a theoretical basis for it – Chadwick believed to the end that infection was due to 'smells' from bad sanitation.

For reforms to take effect, zeal alone is not enough; it must be supplemented by systems for collecting the relevant information, analysing it and setting up a machinery for implementing reforms and later evaluating their effect. The foundations for these matters were also laid in the nineteenth century. The first Act for the Registration of Births and Deaths was passed in 1836; and three years later, in a moment of inspired optimism, the first compiler of statistics was able to say, 'Medicine, like the other natural sciences, is beginning to abandon vague conjecture where facts can accurately be determined by observation; and to substitute numerical expressions for uncertain assertions'. The registration of doctors themselves through the Medical Act of 1858 paved the way for the requirement in 1874 that death certificates should be signed by a registered medical practitioner.

Health authorities, in the form of Boards of Health, were also established, both centrally and locally. A consultative board of health, jointly with the Royal College of Physicians, was set up in 1831, during a cholera epidemic; but a statutory General Board of Health was created following the first Public Health Act in 1848. Local Boards of Health were also established by central authority, but this responsibility was transferred to local government when that evolved in the second half of the century.

THE PRESENT POSITION

Apart from occasional references, I have not attempted any account of the history of medicine in general, for two main reasons. First, the knowledge base and the conditions of practice in therapeutic medicine have changed so radically this century as to make what happened in that area in previous centuries relatively less appropriate to any brief account. Secondly, it would not be reasonable to give even a summary account of the history of general medicine without relating it to the social and even the political history of the various periods, a task far beyond the scope of the present book, let alone my own competence to do it.

Why then have I made an exception by outlining the story of increasing involvement during the past century of both central and local government in the care of the public health?

It is exactly for the reverse of the two reasons I have just given for not attempting an outline of medical history in general. First, the connection between the recent past and the present is closer and more relevant in the public health field than in individual medicine. Secondly, the necessary political background of Parliamentary democracy has remained the same in its main essentials, in spite of great changes such as the extension of the franchise and the increasing recognition of the responsibility of the state for the welfare of its people. A third reason, of course, is that it would be even more difficult to understand the present arrangements for safeguarding the public health without some knowledge of what went before – a complex mix of voluntary and government effort, and within government, of central and local responsibility.

I shall discuss the different possible systems of providing individual health care in the next chapter. All I need say in the present context is that the provision of a National Health Service in 1948 provided an opportunity for linking more closely what had previously been three rather separate areas of medicine – the general practitioner service, which was basically a system of private health care, though there was the Lloyd George insurance scheme for employed persons, initiated in 1911; the hospital service, partly provided by local government, and partly by voluntary effort, the funding of which was becoming precarious; and the public health aspects, partly provided by local authorities with medical officers of health, and partly by central agencies such as the Registrar-General's statistical services. With all the unfairness of a summary statement, it seems to me that the National Health Service has been reasonably successful in raising the standard throughout the country of both general and specialist practice, and has even to some extent succeeded in coordinating these two broad divisions; but the bringing together of individual medicine and public health medicine has not taken place to the same extent.

This relative failure is not due either to lack of administrative effort, or to lack of dedication among those practising in the public health area. Administratively, there was a reorganization of the service in 1974, with the specific objective of unifying the responsibility for the three branches of the service and producing a clear chain of accountability. All that remains of this, following two further attempts at reorganization, is the change of name from 'Regional Hospital Board' to 'Regional Health Authority'. In relation to the actual tasks, concern for the public health has attracted some of the ablest members of the medical profession into that area; moreover, care of the public health, and more attention to preventive medicine, have been fervently advocated both from within the profession and beyond it.

If there has been difficulty in assimilating community medicine (as public health medicine is now often called) to the other branches of medicine, what are the reasons? I can think of three possibilities. At a rather pragmatic level, there is a very considerable *disparity of numbers* between community physicians and those in the other two branches. There are well under 1,000 full-time community physicians, in comparison with some 25,000 general practitioners and around 20,000 hospital doctors; there are, however, some thousands of doctors working on a part-time basis in community clinics, mainly but not exclusively in child health. Secondly, there is a relative lack of drama and urgency about the work of the community physician, which deprives him not only of the glamour of the media (a piece of good fortune which he may not appreciate), but also of the *parity of esteem* which unfair colleagues may accord to those who seem always to be saving lives. Thirdly, at an early stage in the evolution of the specialty of community medicine, it was decided that those engaged in it should not also be involved in the care of individual patients. This represented a change from the days when the medical officer of health had responsibility for the care of patients with infectious diseases. A recent survey showed that about half of the community physicians questioned would have welcomed a clinical involvement. This somewhat artificial *isolation from individual clinical work* can scarcely have assisted integration.

While small numbers, imperfect recognition and isolation from clinical responsibility may have slowed down the progress of community medicine, it would be a grave mistake to regard these factors as in any way undermining the importance of the tasks which community physicians, and their academic colleagues in community medicine, actually perform. Among these tasks are participation in the planning of health services as a whole; planning for the needs of specific groups, such as children, the elderly and the mentally ill and handicapped; developing systems of information for assessing need, and evaluating the efficacy of provision; defining the environmental, social and behavioural determinants of health and disease; controlling communicable diseases, both by prevention and by isolation when necessary; and promoting health education. It must be apparent that these are matters in which community physicians must cooperate not only with other members of their own profession, but also with statisticians, economists, sociologists and professional administrators.

Of these various tasks, I shall leave the ones relating to service provision until the next chapter; and I have already given a general account of the determinants of health and disease in chapters 2 and 3. I can therefore turn to that very important part of community medicine which is concerned with the prevention of ill-health, in the broadest sense.

PREVENTIVE MEDICINE

The prospect of preventing illness, rather than dealing with established illness, is an attractive one, both superficially and at a deeper level. The superficial attraction, enshrined in the proverb, 'Prevention is better than cure', is obvious, and is part of the health policy of all the main political parties. When we go deeper, below the surface of proverbs and political rhetoric, we find there are indeed many encouraging opportunities for practical preventive action. These were convincingly analysed by Sir Richard Doll in his Harveian Oration to the Royal College of Physicians, published in the *British Medical Journal* of 5 February 1983. Great as these opportunities are, however, there are also difficulties, relating to the availability and distribution of resources, and to the public acceptability of preventive measures.

Preventive measures are commonly divided into three categories. *Primary* prevention aims at preventing the occurrence of disease or injury. *Secondary* prevention means early detection of disease, perhaps even before the prospective patient is aware of anything amiss. *Tertiary* prevention aims at minimizing the effects of the disease, and preventing complications. In the case of infective disease, this somewhat artificial wheel comes full circle, since the treatment of the disease (tertiary prevention) may protect other people from acquiring it (primary prevention). I find it rather difficult to distinguish 'tertiary prevention' from the ordinary practice of medicine; and to a lesser extent, the early detection of disease is an important task for the clinician, as well as for the public health doctor. I shall therefore give more attention to the scope for primary prevention, with a short note on screening programmes for the early detection of disease, which are to some extent separable from clinical medicine centred on individuals.

Primary prevention

It is not just a truism to say that the best way to avoid illness is to lead a healthy life in a healthy environment. Put that way, it emphasizes the importance of behavioural and social factors, even, if need be, at the expense of those factors which are 'medical' in a narrow sense, though these also have their importance.

While there is no doubt much still to learn about what makes a 'healthy life-style', the more immediate problem is the imperfect application of what is already known. Smoking tobacco, whether at first or second hand, is a clear health hazard, as is the immoderate consumption of alcohol. Diets which are high in fat and refined carbohydrate, and low in protein and fibre, together with lack of exercise, are the main cause of obesity. One great challenge to health education is to make these simple principles, already largely accepted by the professional classes, better known to the mass of the people. There is, after all, a sensible and enjoyable life available between the extremes of health faddism and indiscriminate self-indulgence. More of us should take advantage of it. It is important, however, not to 'blame the victim' for an illness he may have contracted from thoughtless adherence to the life-style of his social group.

Apart from the behaviour of individuals, there are important social factors in the preservation of health. These are in principle well known – congenial employment, adequate remuneration, proper housing and sanitation, safety in the home and at work, facilities for sport and leisure, and so on. They are not universally available, even in developed countries, and especially in the inner city areas of urban deprivation; and in developing countries they are accessible only to a small minority.

Of course, doctors cannot solve the socioeconomic problems which remove a healthy life-style beyond the reach of millions; but neither should we pretend that these problems do not exist. At the very least, we can be sympathetic to the measures for lessening the effects of unemployment and racial tension in our own country, and bringing clean water and adequate food to the Third World. Although on the global scale behavioural and social influences on health and disease outweigh the strictly medical, there are also important medical initiatives available, which I will now consider.

Control of infection

As already mentioned, effective treatment of infections may also be a preventive measure, by preventing the spread of the infection to other people. A more direct method of prevention is by *inoculation*, the most topical instance of which is the eradication of smallpox from the world nearly 200 years after Jenner introduced the technique of vaccination, published in 1798. *Isolation* of patients with highly infective conditions is another way of containing the spread of infection; and measures of isolation are of course also needed to protect from infection those whose immune mechanisms have been weakened or destroyed by illnesses such as AIDS, or by drugs required to prevent the rejection of transplanted tissue.

As we go through life, and experience various infections, we acquire immunity to them; but if one of these has in the meantime inflicted dangerous illness on us, that is surely worth avoiding. In Britain several thousand children died of diphtheria every year until nationwide immunization was introduced in the 1940s, following which the disease has practically vanished. The production of active immunity by giving a controlled dose of a modified, and thus safe, infective agent has also been effective in poliomyelitis and other serious infections. Although protection of the individual is the most obvious and direct effect of immunization, there is also an advantage to the community, given a sufficient uptake of immunization in the population. Spread of infection depends on a sufficient number of susceptible (non-immune) persons in the population; if the *herd immunity*, achieved by immunizing previously susceptible people, is high enough, the disease cannot spread, and may even die out.

Pollution

Pollution of air, food and water is not controlled by medical means; but medical knowledge is relevant to specifying what pollutants are highly dangerous, and what may be relatively tolerable. Pollution with bacteria and viruses has to be detected using microbiological techniques; but other pollutants are detected by chemical or physical methods, radiation protection being a special and important case. Many important pollutants arise in the course of industrial processes (asbestos, sulphur dioxide, benzine and so on), and are thus of concern to the industrial hygienist and the occupational physician.

Accident

Accidents are an important cause of incapacity and death, especially in children and young people, and again in the elderly. Most accidents occur in the home, due mainly to behavioural factors, but also to overcrowding and faulty design of appliances. Household materials as well as drugs should be shielded from the inquisitiveness of children. Accidents on the roads owe more to bad behaviour than to bad design, but their effects can be lessened by seat-belts and helmets – not medical measures, but owing something to medical advocacy.

Medication

Medicines can be used as preventive agents, for example, iodine in the prevention of cretinism, fluoride in the prevention of dental caries and anti-coagulants to prevent thrombosis.

Screening

Most of the preventive measures so far discussed are relatively uncontroversial in principle, any difficulties arising rather in their practical implementation. Screening pro-grammes are perhaps more difficult to assess, on a cost–benefit basis. They have their advocates, exemplified by this quotation from an American textbook:

Physicians who examine well individuals are not 'wasting their training'. More skill is required to recognize the early signs of ill-health than to deal with what is obvious to patients or their families.

On the other hand, the difficulty of a task, while stimulating, is not a sufficient reason for doing it; and a general screening programme in any sizeable population is a costly undertaking. More important, the value of *general* or *global* screening is by no means proved. One study in

London has indicated no difference in the five-year survival of patients subjected to annual screening compared with random unscreened controls from the same group of practices. A Canadian review, after careful analysis, suggested that the 'annual check-up' be abandoned.

On the other hand, screening for specific conditions (which must be treatable!) at the time of life when they are liable to occur, is worth while; for example, taking the blood pressure as a routine in older people, screening for breast or cervical cancer in women, and so on. In these specific screening programmes, it is important that there should be firm criteria of diagnosis; not only intrinsic treatability, but also available facilities to carry it out; and a good communication system, with particular attention to preventing any anxiety about the programme itself. Ante-natal examination of the mother is clearly important, to identify obstetric risk factors and to detect serious fetal anomalies. Paediatric examination is also important, to detect correctable congenital defects.

Mention of ante-natal screening provides an opportunity to say something of a condition which illustrates rather well the point that prevention and cure are not locked in separate compartments, but can be used as parts of a coordinated programme. The condition is beta-thalassaemia, also known as Cooley's anaemia; it is an inherited disorder more common in the Levant than elsewhere. The mode of inheritance is as an autosomal recessive gene (see chapter 2), so that if two carriers marry, they have a 50 per cent chance of producing another carrier, a 25 per cent chance of producing an affected infant and a 25 per cent chance of producing a completely normal child. In an affected infant, one or other form of abnormal haemoglobin is produced, and the red cells have a short lifespan. The condition is serious, with an expectation of life of only a few years if no treatment is given. Life can be materially prolonged by blood transfusion, but the body is unable to get rid of the iron being added to it by repeated transfusions, and this accumulates in organs such as the liver, causing damage and ultimate liver failure. This complication in turn can be controlled by giving desferrioxamine, which binds the iron in a soluble form which can then be excreted; but this substance has to be given by subcutaneous infusion over several hours, and repeatedly, so the treatment itself is a strain, although well worth it in terms of prolongation and quality of life.

The alternative approach is prevention, though the term is something of a euphemism, as it involves the loss of an affected fetus. Here again, fundamental work in molecular biology has brought about a practical advance, in that it is now possible, using radioactive probes, to carry out direct gene analysis on biopsy specimens of the fetal component of the developing placenta a few weeks after the start of pregnancy. Before this advance, detection of the abnormal haemoglobin produced by the defective gene could not be achieved until around the eighteenth week of pregnancy. The much earlier stage at which an abnormal fetus can now be diagnosed makes termination possible at a time when it is easier and less distasteful. There is, of course, no point in undertaking these investigations if the parents are opposed to termination; but it is of interest that the proportion of affected infants born to carrier parents in parts of Italy where the disease is common is very much lower than in the Cypriot community in this country. This suggests that even in Italy pregnancy is being either prevented or terminated.

I have given this example at some length to show the complexity of the issues that have to be laid before parents known to be carrying a harmful hereditary trait; but even more to underline the interdependence of treatment and prevention, and also the relevance of fundamental studies, such as in molecular biology here, to the actual practice of medicine.

8

Providing Health Care

I have now given at some length an outline of how individuals may benefit from medical care, and more briefly how medical knowledge can be applied to the general health of populations. In primitive societies, medical care is provided at the village level, and needs no more organization than knowing where a suitable healer, shaman or witch-doctor is to be found. The development which we call civilization greatly extends the range of possible benefits; but this brings with it the need to devise some kind of system so that what is possible can be made actual to the greatest extent that resources permit. In this way, a variety of systems of health care have come into being, with interesting differences in different countries, and even in different parts of the same country. Before looking at the types of system which have arisen, it may be worth sparing a little time to consider what are the legitimate aims of a health care system.

AIMS OF A HEALTH SERVICE

Some commentators have considered that priority should be given to the advancement of science, and particularly of medical science; to the preservation of life, and particularly human life, at whatever cost; or to the benefit of society as a whole, even if this entails considerable hardship to individuals. These are all worthwhile aims, but to no one of them would I personally assign the highest priority. I hope that in the earlier part of this book I made sufficiently clear my belief in the importance of medical science and its advancement; but this should not be the chief aim of a health care system. Again, to elevate the preservation of life to the station of an absolute principle, especially when codified on a legal basis, entails such consequences as preserving an unconscious patient for years on end, and burdening families with handicapped children destined to misery which they themselves are scarcely capable of comprehending, but which cause great distress to their anxious parents who wonder what will happen to the children when they themselves have gone. Thirdly, society, like chance, is a fine thing, but I personally believe that society was made for (and by) man, and not man for society; or to put it more plainly, individual welfare is a necessary component of the just society.

Underlying my doubts over giving a top priority to one of these three reasonable-seeming aims, is my consciousness of the danger of applying general principles to every individual situation. Secondly, I believe these matters, important as they are, are tangential to the main purposes of a health care system, which are to care for those who are ill, curing them if possible; to maintain the health of the people, both by general and by specific measures; and to do these things in a way which is consistent with the welfare of those providing the various forms of care.

I find it difficult to assign priorities between these three aims of a health service. I have in fact arranged them in order of descending priority, as I would judge it, but I also believe that they cannot reasonably be dissociated. Even the third of them, the welfare of workers in the service, while it can be represented as 'selfish', is an important foundation for a service of quality. If staff of all or any grade are discontented, this will lower the quality of the service which they give. Again, the maintenance of health almost by definition contributes to alleviating the burden of illness. It is all very well for cynics critical of prevention to say that the burden of illness is not prevented, only postponed to strike more heavily in a decrepit old age. Such an argument ignores even the economic value of the labour of those who have been preserved from premature illness, bringing disability or death; but also the human value of added years of healthy life.

Why then do I still give the highest priority to the actual care of the sick – a judgement which runs contrary to a great deal of sociological and political thinking? I do so on grounds of urgency, preferring a close and visible type of need to one, however important, which is distant and perhaps theoretical. The distant scene should not be an excuse for neglecting the task which lies to hand; Blake had a wise word when he said, 'He who would do good to another must do it in Minute Particulars'. I would perhaps be more hesitant to follow him when he goes on to say, 'General Good is the plea of the scoundrel, hypocrite and flatterer'. To go so far blurs the common ground between 'preventive' and 'curative' medicine. Just as good prevention lessens the burden of illness and the need for treatment, so effective treatment of acute conditions prevents the development of chronic disability.

CONSTRAINTS ON HEALTH CARE

My view of the objectives of a health care system in a developed country is a personal one, but one which I believe would be shared by the majority of practising doctors. Before I go on to describe actual systems, it is important to look at the types of constraint which have to be overcome in developing an ideal service. These constraints relate in part to the availability and deployment of resources; in part to the ways in which information is gathered and used; and in perhaps the largest part to the attitudes of those who provide the service, and to a lesser extent, those who use it. These various forms of constraint need not be described here in detail, but it may be worth giving some indication of what I mean.

Economic constraints

These arise both at the national, even the global, level of 'macro-economics' and also in relation to the myriad individual decisions of 'micro-economics'.

To take the national level first, there is general agreement that even the wealthiest countries, which tend also to be the countries that spend the highest proportion of their gross national product on health-related expenditure, are nevertheless falling short of meeting the total need. How much more must this be true of the poorest countries, which spend less on health not only absolutely but proportionately. Recognition of the 'open-endedness' of health expenditure has come rather slowly, and perhaps the first Minister of Health to enunciate it clearly was Dr David Owen. With a gross national product per head much smaller than that in the USA, we in the UK spend about 6 per cent of our GNP on health, while the USA spends more than 10 per cent. It is hard to say whether we are getting a good bargain from having in the main a state health service, or whether we are being unduly niggardly – perhaps both.

At the micro-economic level, the aim – not, I hasten to say, realized – is to achieve a balance between particular needs, the demands to which they give rise and the provision of resources to meet the demands. In an ideal world, the prime determinant of provision should be the actual need for it; but in the real world, irrespective of the nature of the system, what is provided, within the general constraints of what can be afforded, depends more on demand than on need, and may even be largely independent of both, and determined by the choices of professional providers or managers. In spite of what is often believed, actual surveys show that there are many health needs stemming from illnesses perceived as minor which never give rise to any demands on the health services; and to a much lesser extent, demands occur which do not relate to any easily discernible need. A similar discrepancy can sometimes be observed between what is required or asked for and what is provided; there may even be some excuse for this, based on the wastefulness of making provision for all contingencies, of which the majority may never happen. Perhaps I can illustrate this last point obliquely, from an actual experience many years ago which perhaps set me thinking on these lines. I was intrigued to see, in what was then Bengal, a local doctor giving another Indian an intravenous injection. I asked him what he was doing, and he said, 'I am giving him calcium'. Pursuing my arrogant course, I asked him, 'Why?', and got the answer, 'Calcium is all I have got'.

Constraints related to information

One of the obvious constraints imposed by the type of information relevant to health care is the sheer bulk of it, arising from the large number of individuals from whom it has to be derived. Although the ultimate use of the information may not require that any individual be identified, the accuracy of any conclusions will be lost if at the stage of gathering information there is not precise identification of the individual to whom it relates. With unusual names this may be no great problem, but what of the Joneses and Smiths, and more recently the Mahomeds. Simply for identification purposes, additional information such as date of birth or mother's maiden name has to be recorded.

A reliable patient index imposes quite a burden on either manual or machine data systems. The coming of mechanical data-processing – not merely computers but also software specialized for health information requirements – has helped both the storage and the analysis of health information, though at some cost, both in the sophistication of apparatus and in the level of skill demanded of those who are engaged in data-processing.

In addition to the bulk of health information, there is the constraint imposed by the need for confidentiality, already mentioned in chapter 6. The necessary protection of personal health information from those who do *not* need access to it entails some restriction of the ease with which those who *do* need to know it can be given access to it.

Quite apart from the problem set by the need to hold information on individual patients in any organized system, there is the problem set by the rapid expansion of the amount of knowledge which is relevant to patient care. There is talk in all the sciences of 'the information explosion', and medical science is not only no exception to this, but perhaps an extreme example. One response to this has been increased specialization; but even in a restricted area of medicine the specialist has to consult with colleagues, to study textbooks and increasingly to have either direct or postal access to data-bases on disc or tape.

Information of different types is also needed for the quality control of the services provided, and for assessing the priorities of various possible areas of service. It is all too easy to gather discrete nuggets of information as a squirrel gathers nuts; but the value of information depends not on its amount, but on its usefulness, and this implies critical analysis. For example, a low figure for bed-occupancy on a surgical ward is not a good reason for bringing in patients to be operated on Monday on the preceding Friday, rather than the Sunday evening before.

There may also be a risk of reaching wrong conclusions if too much reliance is placed on a single index of priority, when several are available. Some years ago, a colleague and I worked out the 'burden' on the health service arising from about 50 broad categories of disease, such as infection, peptic ulcer, tumours, bronchitis and so on. We used five indices: hospital bed occupation; outpatient visits; visits to a family doctor; payments for sickness benefit; and mortality, expressed as loss of life expectancy, in order to bring it nearer to economic terms. There were notable differences between the conclusions we could have drawn from the different indices. For example, about half of the burden on hospital beds arose from mental illness and handicap; whereas over half the loss of life-expectancy was accounted for by heart disease and tumours. Other indices showed less extreme differences in their profile of burden. At the end of this road, definition of priorities still requires a value judgement, to answer questions such as, 'Do we want to cut down on hospital beds?', in which case we could direct resources to mental illness, or 'Do we want to prolong useful life?', in which case we devote more effort to the prevention and care of heart attacks. But at the very least this type of analysis, tedious as it may seem, offers an alternative approach to the competitive rhetoric of the pressure groups who champion particular disease states, some of them rather uncommon.

Constraints arising from attitudes

Modern health care is a complex activity, bringing together a range of professional disciplines and also a large staff of ancillary workers. It would be surprising if members of these various professions and groups did not occasionally overlook their common duty to the service, and indulge either as individuals or collectively in disputes with authority or in interprofessional rivalries. In speaking of communication, I have already recognized that while doctors may have a longer training than the majority of health professionals, these also have important and particular skills. Similarly, revolt against authority is by no means necessarily entirely the fault of those engaged in it.

This said, however, I must nevertheless state my own view that anything approaching 'withdrawal of labour', or setting the status of the profession over the need for teamwork, is a disaster. The remedy, easy to say but difficult always to remember in situations of stress, is that all engaged in the health service must remind themselves of the chief purpose of the whole enterprise, without which all else is pointless – the need to help patients in whatever way is appropriate, be it prevention, cure or care.

Of course, in the real world it may be impossible to meet all the wishes and needs of a patient and his relatives, and this is another possible cause of attitudinal strain. To say that 'the patient should come first' is not quite the same thing as to say, 'the patient (or a relative) is always right'. A patient's autonomy is a vital possession, but his right to it is not absolute, should he become incapable of exercising it, for mental or physical reasons. In such a case, and being careful to achieve the understanding and consent of relatives whenever possible, the doctor or other health professional has to act as proxy for the patient. The essential safeguard is that as effective autonomy returns in the course of recovery, the doctor must be anxious to withdraw from the paternalistic role which has been thrust upon him. Paternalism is at times a necessary drug, but it has side-effects on the person who exercises it, as well as on the sufferer.

There is one further possible cause of constraint between doctors and their patients, which is difficult to describe, but I believe it to be real, and at times material. The conventional picture of illness embraces the stereotypes of the cheerful and long-suffering patient, and the caring doctor, nurse and so on. But the facts have also to be faced that on the one hand illness is an unpleasant experience, capable of making people behave unreasonably, and on the other hand, doctors and nurses can be tired and under emotional strain, and at times under par.

Just as in ordinary life different people are more or less pleasant to meet, similarly medical practitioners, being human, warm to some patients more than to others. Even so, one must always keep in mind the disturbing effect of perceived illness on anyone, and make suitable allowance. Some illnesses, and not only primarily mental illnesses, can of course lead to behaviour which seriously strains the patience of the most tolerant individual. Examples of 'non-mental' behaviour disorders, known collectively as 'the organic dementias', include the delirium of high fever, the disturbed behaviour seen in advanced kidney or liver failure, the effect of drugs, including alcohol, and the dullness of hypothyroidism, which may sometimes break out into 'myxoedema madness'. Recognition of these and other forms of dementia is important, not only because some of them are remediable, but also because it prevents something being attributed to a patient's basic personality which really a part of his illness.

However, even when all allowance has been made for the effects of illness, there are some basic characteristics of personality which can affect the meeting between patient and doctor adversely. They are by no means all on one side, but for the moment we are dealing with patients. One American doctor (whose first name was Solomon, but he may not have shared the wisdom of his forebear) was brave enough to describe several categories of 'the undesirable patient'. These include (and I emphasize that I am quoting), 'the ungrateful and obnoxious', those with untreatable illness, or at the other extreme those with no discoverable illness, and 'those who are undesirable because the physician considers them to be a distraction to preferred tasks, such as reading or laboratory research'. Some of these descriptions seem to reflect at least as much on the doctor as on the patient, the last of them particularly indicating a lack of dedication to clinical practice. Without going quite so far, I would be willing to admit that some patients draw more liberally than others on the reservoir of patience which should be at every practising doctor's command.

Turning to the weaknesses of doctors, some of them are excusable on grounds of tiredness, overwork, emotional stress and, in the younger doctors, anxiety about examinations and career prospects, together with long hours of duty and increasing responsibilities. These are possible excuses, but not justifications for impatience in dealing with clinical problems. What cannot ever be justified whatever the provocation, is rudeness to patients, and when it occurs it is more often the basis of a complaint than is lack of clinical judgement. The public rightly expect a high ethical standard from doctors, and increasingly they should expect a high standard of up-to-date knowledge. In this context, the high quality of students entering medicine, and the development of training programmes and refresher courses should make the ignorant and out-dated doctor even rarer in the future than he is now. Knowledge, of course, is not enough by itself; to be effective in practice it has to be supplemented by kindness and a sense of duty. One important component of medical ethics which sometimes escapes mention in text-books devoted to the subject is the duty a doctor has, first to become competent at his job, and then to maintain that competence in line with advances in knowledge and practice.

Having considered then the objectives of a health service, and some of the constraints which may hinder their attainment, it is time to look at some of the patterns of provision which have developed to meet these needs.

SYSTEMS OF HEALTH CARE

For the greatest part of the long history of medicine, the care of the sick was handled very largely on an informal basis, in classical times by the priesthood or even by slaves. Even after a recognizable profession had developed, trained in universities and licensed in various ways by corporations, the greater part of medical care was still given by wise women, quacks of various kinds and so on. For any recognizable system of health care to appear, it was necessary for doctors, nurses and other health workers to be identifiable by registration, and also to be charged with the responsibility for giving the preponderance of health care. The responsibility of professionals for giving health care has never been complete, and never will be. The greatest number of episodes of minor illness, and some which are not so minor, are either borne by the patient himself, or cared for by relatives, friends or occasionally unqualified people. But until a hundred years ago or even less, medical attention given by qualified doctors was limited to the rich and famous, or to those poorer people who could be recommended for admission to a charitable hospital either by a patron or because of the severity of their illness. Moreover, even if medicine was something of a luxury, those who paid for it did not always get a good bargain – not because doctors then were particularly stupid or covetous, but because they lacked the knowledge to discern what was worth doing, and they were also lumbered by tradition with dangerous and ineffective procedures such as blood-letting and purgation. To be a member of a royal family was particularly dangerous. The last illness of Charles II was a nightmare, especially for a man who when in health had said to a friend, 'I would not have you take overmuch physic, for it doth alway make me the worse, and it may do the like with you'. Louis XIV of France was succeeded by his great-grandson, the intermediate heirs having been disposed of by the court physician Fagon, whose advice was mandatory for all but the king himself.

I am not, of course, suggesting that our present-day knowledge of medicine is complete. Far from it, and many challenges of ignorance remain. But this century has seen a real transformation towards a general diffusion of practically useful medical knowledge and away from the days when in spite of the intellect and dedication of doctors there was really little they could do to improve actual outcomes of illness, and indeed much that was done could be harmful. As one cynic said, there was not much difference between good medicine and no medicine at all, but a lot of difference between good medicine and bad medicine. There are, of course, many diseases for which this would still be true; but the happy thing is that effective treatments are now available for a great number of conditions that were untreatable 50 years ago. There is no reason to suppose that the methods of research and development which have been successful in the past will suddenly lose all their virtue, even though the remaining problems may seem intractable in the light of present knowledge.

In contrast to past times, there is now an appreciation in developed countries that some system of health care is both necessary and desirable. This has come about for a number of reasons. At the risk of professional arrogance, I would put at the head a general recognition that medical care, whether preventive or curative, is something of real value. From this two things follow: it should be administered by properly qualified people, and it should be available to all who need it. The first of these matters became possible when members of the relevant professions not only underwent training, but had their qualifications registered; the second stemmed from the egalitarian impulse which was calling increasingly into question the rigid stratification of mediaeval society, even though it was not embodied in constitutional form until

American independence and the French revolution. Practical implementation does not necessarily follow the recognition of a principle with any indecent haste. The ideas that medical help was worth having, and that it should be generally available, were around for a considerable time before they were made available to the general employed population, on an insurance basis, in the Lloyd George Act of 1911; and another quarter-century was to pass before a National Health Service was made available to the entire population in 1948. There is one other prerequisite for a system of health care which should be mentioned – there must be a sufficient apparatus of central and local administration for the system to be made effective.

Within the framework of belief that a system of health care is desirable, there is still plenty of room for debate on the detail of how it should be provided. I shall mention only two of these areas of possible debate: how health care should be paid for, and how the system should be administered.

Professional health care is not a free good, like fresh air or sunshine; someone has to pay for it. The main possible options are payment out of general taxation, payment by individual insurance and direct payment by individuals to doctors. None of these systems excludes the others, and in general they co-exist.

The major issue is between state provision and private provision, whether by insurance or by fee for service. Many people see this as an issue of principle, perhaps even of prejudice. State provision appeals to those who assign top priority to fair play and egalitarianism; private provision to those who emphasize individual freedom and responsibility. I believe the extremes of equality and of liberty should both be tempered by fraternity and I follow the Merrison Royal Commission in the general view that the most economical way of providing a medical service is from general taxation, but that a minority private sector is admissible. There seems to me to have been a general consensus on these lines in this country; and the health service has brought a generally acceptable standard of health care to all parts of our country in a way that would have been difficult to achieve by a privately financed system. We have also been fortunate in retaining a strong system of general practice, providing primary care directly and also acting as a gateway to the specialist services. That these matters may look somewhat different from the other side of the Atlantic was brought home to me some years ago when I was talking to an American lady at a party. She said, 'Have you gotten penicillin in your socialized health service?'. I took some pleasure in telling her some relevant recent medical history from St Mary's where penicillin was first observed and Oxford where it was made effective. There is in all countries a gap between the best and the worst medical provision and this is perhaps wider in the USA than in the UK, partly because the best in the USA is so good.

Another matter of some importance, and also some topicality, relates to the manner in which decisions should be made in an organized system. There is a tension between central control and local autonomy, in which a reasonable balance may have been achieved; but there is more controversy at present about the style of management. One view, which has prevailed until fairly recently, is that the really important decisions are those which affect the patients, and that these are best made by the professionals entrusted with their care – not only the doctors, but the various professional groups involved, including the administrator. This sort of system is known as 'consensus management'. The alternative, at present in vogue in this country, draws its inspiration from business management, and has led to the appointment of 'general managers' at the various levels of the health service. This does have the advantage that it is easy to identify, and hold to account a particular individual, who thus has an inducement to see that all goes well. I do not think, however, that it is merely professional bias which makes me, together with many of my colleagues both in medicine and in nursing, have a strong preference for consensus management, which worked very well in the first 30 years of the service. Looking after people in health and in illness seems to me a very different operation from selling sugar or making cars. The search for people to come in from the business world to 'run the health service' brings in a new principle of recruitment, that ignorance of the problem is a qualification for filling a post. Not surprisingly, the quest has been none too successful. As an optimist, I hope that the injection of commercial management into health service administration may be a passing phase, and that consensus management will be restored.

In conclusion, however, let me say that even important matters such as the methods of payment and administration are ultimately of less importance than the quality and availability of a service. Methods of payment and administration influence a service at the margin, but the really important matter is the dedication of those who work in it, determined to make that service a success for the welfare of people and patients.

9

Medicine and Society

A few years ago I drew attention to a paradox of opinion relating to modern medicine, outlining it in these words: 'Whereas the potential of medical knowledge for preserving and restoring health has never been greater, the systems for applying it have never been so sharply criticised'. In this book, I have tried to describe the nature of medical knowledge and its application both to individual problems and to the health of the people as a whole. I believe the record of modern medicine to be both true and good in its essentials, whatever the shortcomings of individual practitioners (and which of us is free from error at times?). But in this concluding chapter I want to consider some of the general criticisms being made of medicine at this time, and if possible to rebut them. In order to give a general view to begin with, I shall summarize some of the statements made, or beliefs held, about medicine, and then go on to consider them individually. Being a doctor, I may give undue emphasis to criticisms made of doctors, but I recognize that the more general criticisms apply also to nurses and indeed to all who work in health care.

Criticism comes from various sources – publicists, sociologists, lawyers, economists and, not least, doctors and nurses themselves. Without particular attribution, I shall draw from these various sources to give a general summary of what is said in criticism of present-day health care. Such a summary might go something like this:

Medicine today is excessively preoccupied with science and the technology which stems from the scientific approach; this dehumanizes doctors and nurses, so that they see the body as a set of parts [some use the disturbing analogy that they see it as a garage mechanic sees a car]. Because of this, care of the whole person is lost, and also doctors may become 'agents of society', whether the ends of a particular society are good or bad. Doctors and nurses rob the patient of his autonomy, not just by prolonging life, but also by relieving pain, which according to Ivan Illich is not only a necessary but actually a valuable part of life. Doctors and nurses spend time and effort in the study and attempted cure of rare diseases, whereas they should be concentrating much more on prevention, and on the care of chronic illness, especially as it affects particular groups, such as the elderly. In any case, the whole enterprise is rather a waste of resources, as the real causes of ill-health are social and psychological.

Of course, not every critic of medicine would make all these criticisms, while some critics are not even consistent. I well remember one occasion when a doctor holding some of these views, and allocated 15 minutes in which to express them, devoted 15 minutes to explaining why medicine was useless, and a further 15 minutes to complaining that medicine was not equally available to all social classes. Nevertheless, these criticisms must be taken seriously, as they have been given wide currency in the media and may be in part responsible for the current vogue for non-scientifically based forms of therapy. By answering them, I hope to convince you that the type of medicine currently available is a social good, and a career in medicine is justifiable and indeed valuable.

The first question to be addressed is whether present-day medicine is useful, first to the individual and then to society.

So far as the individual is concerned, most critics would concede that there are some conditions in which soundly based diagnosis and treatment are of benefit to the patient. However, some critics would go on to say that the illness should have been prevented in the first place; and others will point to the many conditions for which there is still no effective answer. Both these reservations are valid, but to

190

admit them should not be an excuse for complacency, but rather a spur to further effort to learn more about preventive measures, and to extend the scope of effective treatment to those diseases for which it is still not available. It is unfortunate that the benefits of modern medicine do not include immortality; but for many individuals, though not of course for all, there are hosts of ways in which the correct application of skilled diagnosis followed by appropriate treatment can restore quality of life to a sufferer from chronic invalidism, or prevent a death which without modern therapy would have been inevitable.

For my own part I would be well content to base the 'defence' of modern medicine on what it can do for particular individuals. But this will not satisfy those who regard the welfare of society as a greater good than the welfare of individuals. (Myself, I think these two things rather go together.) The main sociological criticism is twofold, that doctors and nurses as a group are neglectful of social issues and the particular needs of 'client groups'; and that their concentration on the individual makes their commitment to overall health a marginal one at best.

The first of these charges (neglect of broad social issues) is to a limited extent true; most doctors are fully occupied in a very absorbing responsibility, that of caring for individual patients. But even the busiest clinical doctor must be aware of the social background from which his patients come, provided of course that he takes a normal human interest in them – and in spite of the critics, I believe that is what the great majority of doctors do, and certainly all those who enjoy what might be called clinical success. The speechless doctor who sticks tubes into you is unlikely to enjoy the respect of his colleagues and patients for long. Over and above the general social awareness which I would be willing to ascribe to those engaged in actual clinical practice, however, I would draw attention to the considerable number of doctors engaged in what may be called 'the medicine of populations', whether these be geographically defined, or defined by specific occupations, or by belonging to particular 'client groups' (so-called – I would prefer 'patient' to 'client') such as pregnant women, children or the elderly. Social awareness is at the very centre of the responsibilities of the community physician and the occupational physician, who form an important part of the medical profession.

Let me now turn to the more fundamental sociological criticism shared by many doctors, and indeed again a partial truth, that the main causes of disease are social and psychological rather than physical, from which it follows that diagnosis and treatment based on the 'hard sciences' are rather beside the point. According to this view, effort should be directed not towards medicine, but to social preventive measures, such as control of tobacco and other addictive drugs; to better housing and other aspects of the relief of poverty, and so on. I have, of course, stressed in earlier chapters that these are all matters of the first importance in relation to health, but it is just as important to remember that they are not the whole story by any means. Difficulty in forming a judgement on this matter stems from the obvious consideration that improvements in social conditions and improvements in medical knowledge commonly go together, at any rate during the past half-century; it thus becomes a matter of speculation which is the more important, and by how much the more important, in determining any improvement in health.

Even those critics who acknowledge the value of modern medicine for the health of individuals, nevertheless tend to discount its value for populations, in spite of such things as the eradication of smallpox. A typical statement is, 'The therapeutic advances of the past four decades have had little effect on death rates'. How little is 'little'? The answer to that important question must depend on studies of mortality over time, including both general mortality and mortality from particular diseases. We have at the present time some diseases for which medical treatments are available, and others for which there is still no effective treatment; let us call the first group 'amenable' and the second 'non-amenable'. We can now look at two recent studies suggesting that medical treatment may have played a rather larger part in the decline of population mortality than has been conventionally believed.

One study* was based on mortality figures from 1951 to 1980 in England and Wales, Sweden, Italy, France, Japan and USA. Not too surprisingly, in each of these countries the fall in mortality from 'amenable' diseases was substantially greater than that from all other causes. For example, between 1956 and 1978 in England and Wales, for people between 5 and 64 years of age, mortality from 'amenable causes' fell from 68.6 per 100,000 to 33.4 per 100,000; while that from 'all other causes' fell only from 327.2 per 100,000 to 313.0 per 100,000. The authors of this study acknowledged changes in social and other factors which they had not examined, but they still concluded, with proper caution, that 'the consistency in mortality trends for this group of "amenable" diseases suggested that improvements in medical care were a factor in their rapid decline'. It has, of course, to be recognized that deaths from 'non-amenable causes' considerably exceed those from 'amenable causes', so that for overall mortality the effect of rapid decline in the 'amenable' cases is diluted by the larger number of deaths still occurring in the 'non-amenable' group. Thus, a direct comparison of a 51 per cent decline in 'amenable deaths' with a 4 per cent decline in 'non-amenable deaths' overstates the case for the significance of medical intervention. A fairer measure might be the percentage ratio of 'amenable' to 'total' deaths in 1956 and 1978 respectively, which comes out at 17 per cent and 10 per cent.

Another study† from Finland, considered mortality over a shorter period (1969–81). The findings were qualitatively similar, but the authors analysed them in a somewhat different way. 'Amenable mortality' fell by 63 per cent in

---

* Charlton, R. H. and Velez, R. Some international comparisons of mortality amenable to medical intervention. *British Medical Journal* 1986; *1*, 295–301.

† Poikolainen, K. and Eskola, J. The effect of health services on mortality: decline in death rates from amenable and non-amenable causes in Finland, 1969–1981. *Lancet* 1986; *1*, 199–202.

men and 68 per cent in women; while 'non-amenable mortality' fell by 24 per cent and 29 per cent respectively. The time course of the decline in male mortality is shown in figure 3. The authors took the fall of 'non-amenable mortality' as a measure of the effect of social factors and on this basis suggest that the effect of medical measures is indicated by the difference between the 'amenable' and 'non-amenable' rates. This has the weakness that social factors might not necessarily have the same effect on the two groups of diseases.

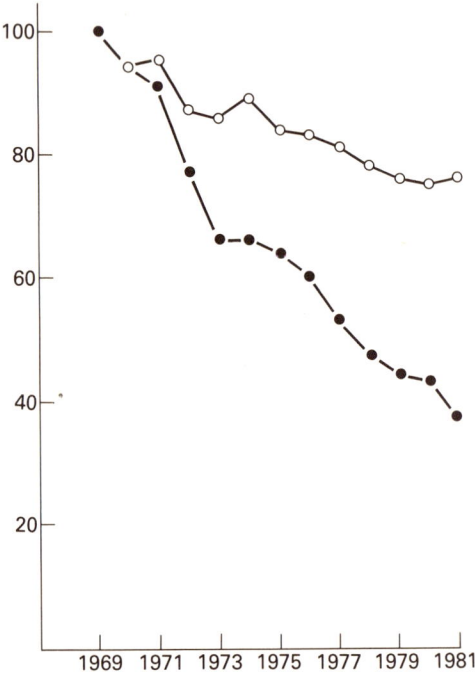

Figure 3 Mortality of males in Finland over the period 1969–81, from diseases 'amenable' to treatment (●—●), and from diseases 'non-amenable' to treatment (o—o). The points from each year are expressed as a percentage of the 1969 figure, which was 47 per 100,000 population for 'amenable' diseases, and 222 per 100,000 population for 'non-amenable' diseases.

Taking the two studies together, however, there is at least a suggestion that medical interventions may be of similar importance to general social factors, a conclusion which perhaps involves no more assumptions than were made in the analyses, stretching back into the last century for data, which would ascribe only a very limited importance to medical interventions. I hope I have supplied at least some grounds for my firm belief that medical services are, on balance, a benefit both to individuals and to society.

Analyses based on mortality can show only a part of the picture, even though such analyses have the advantage of quantification based on a definite event. But modern medicine also has effects on the quality of life. In an imperfect world, however, not all of these are good – modern surgical procedures and modern medicines are potent, but their very potency carries a risk of complications and side-effects. By their nature, these affect individuals, and it is not possible to 'put a figure' on these on a population basis, as can be done with tallies of mortality. But to give a fair perspective it must also be said that the benefits of modern medicine are by no means limited to averting or postponing death. In my view improved quality of life is at least as important, and it is being achieved daily not only by medicines for the relief of pain, sickness and depression, but also by surgical procedures, of which hip replacement is perhaps the most clear-cut and notable example.

The final line of criticism to which I will turn admits at any rate some of the usefulness of scientific medicine, but regards its ministers (the doctors and to a lesser extent the nurses) as being blinded by science and technology, arrogant and paternalistic at one and the same time and incapable of understanding patients as people. The sooner medicine can be rescued from such people, runs this view, the better.

It is, of course, good that our backs should be chastened with such rods from time to time; and they reinforce that humility which every decent doctor should feel in face of the mysteries of life and death. But I do not feel it is really necessary that he should share all his dilemmas with the patient; and if he is never willing to pretend to a show of self-confidence which he may not actually feel, he may be neglecting an important form of treatment. Among their ranks, doctors number some who are arrogant, some who are paternalistic and some who are altruistic, while the same person may be all three of these at different times. I believe, in distinction to many sociologists who have written on the subject, that the majority of doctors both feel themselves to be, and in fact are, on the side of the patient – they would be fools if they were not, for on what else does the practice of medicine ultimately depend? Of course, we can all of us slip from proper standards, but the pressures from patients, from colleagues and from society at large all work in the direction of persuading us to conform to high standards.

Also, an individual sense of duty is supported by a broad consensus of professional ethics, backed up by the esteem of colleagues and, if necessary, by the discipline of health authorities, of the General Medical Council and of the courts. There have been various codifications of medical ethics, and a proliferation of textbooks, but the real safeguards are love of mankind, love of the art and love of the knowledge needed to practise it.

As I conclude this attempt to depict a complex scene with a broad brush on a restricted canvas, I am conscious of both unavoidable bias and incompleteness. My bias is that of a general physician, which may have made me give too much stress to the organic aspects of disease, however much I may have noted the importance of psychological and social factors. I have many friends in all branches of the profession but it remains true that had I been a family doctor, or a surgeon, or a psychiatrist, I would have written a different book. But I have at least tried to emphasize things which are common to all branches of medicine – the conjunction of scientific knowledge and personal skills, the interaction between individual make-up and environmental advantages or strains, and the combination of altruism and firmness which is needed to support the joys and sorrows of medical practice.

Let me now end as I began, with an assurance to prospective students that if you have some 'feel' for science and if you want to help people, or even society, and if what I have told you, or you have heard elsewhere, of medicine interests you, then you should think seriously of choosing first medicine, and later one of its many branches, for your life's work. Should you make that choice, the practicalities of getting into a medical school have been well set out in *Learning Medicine* by Professor Peter Richards, Dean of St Mary's Hospital Medical School, published by the British Medical Association, 1983.

Further Reading

Having come thus far, you will now appreciate that the amount of information which a medical student must acquire is considerable; and further that its acquisition is not a once-for-all achievement, but merely the start of a life-long process of revision, made necessary by the speed with which relevant medical knowledge increases. From time to time, as in any active science, what appeared to be established has to be discarded, or at any rate radically altered or set in a new context. It follows that the basic textbooks appropriate for a medical student have later to be supplemented by monographs dealing with particular areas of medical knowledge; by a very extensive periodical literature, which can disseminate new knowledge more rapidly than the textbook or monograph; and even by frequently revised computer programs. My suggestions for further reading will be illustrative, and not comprehensive; and it is unlikely that you will want to read more than a few of the monographs mentioned, dealing with particular areas. I shall, however, try to mention at least one textbook dealing with the divisions of medical knowledge outlined in the successive chapters of this book, such as genetics and immunology among basic sciences, and public health and medical ethics at the 'applied' end of the spectrum. I have not generally given dates of publication, as the latest edition should always be sought.

Further Reading

In this section I give widely used and often long-established textbooks for the main subjects of the undergraduate medical course. Most medical schools supply a list of 'recommended textbooks', but as I am writing for the general reader what follows is a personal selection.

Anatomy

Cunningham's Textbook of Anatomy, ed. G. J. Romanes (Oxford University Press).

Gray's Anatomy, ed. R. Warwick and P. L. Williams (Longmans).

These are both standard books on the structure of the body. A book that portrays both structure (anatomy) and function (physiology) in the same volume, and which is attractively illustrated, is

Principles of Anatomy and Physiology, G. J. Tortora and N. P. Anagostokos (Harper & Row).

Physiology

Textbook of Medical Physiology, A. C. Guyton (Saunders).

Biochemistry

Essentials of Human Biochemistry. C. R. Paterson (Pitman).

Pathology

Muir's Textbook of Pathology, J. R. Anderson (Arnold).

Microbiology

Medical Microbiology, R. F. Boyd and J. J. Marr (Little, Brown).

Pharmacology

Clinical Pharmacology, R. H. Girdwood (Baillière Tindall).

This is a well reputed student textbook, but for a more compendious insight into the therapeutic revolution, one of the outstanding contemporary textbooks is

The Pharmacological Basis of Therapeutics, A. G. Gilman, L. S. Goodman and A. Gilman (Macmillan).

In all these subjects, which form the mainstream of basic medical knowledge, there is a wide choice of appropriate textbooks, and the above selection is arbitrary. The difficulty becomes still greater when we pass on to clinical subjects – medicine, surgery, obstetrics, paediatrics and psychiatry, and I shall mention only the general textbooks here, leaving monographs till later.

Medicine

Oxford Textbook of Medicine, D. J. Weatherall, J. G. G. Ledingham and D. A. Warrell (Oxford University Press).
Davidson's Principles and Practice of Medicine, J. Macleod (Churchill Livingstone).
Cecil Textbook of Medicine, P. B. Beeson and J. B. Wyngaarden (Saunders).
The Principles and Practice of Medicine, A. M. Harvey, R. J. Johns, V. A. McKusick, A. H. Owens and R. S. Ross (Appleton, Century, Crofts).
Coming from Scotland, *Davidson* is naturally the shortest of these tomes, and thus more popular with students, but the others are meatier.

Surgery

Bailey & Love's Short Practice of Surgery, A. J. Harding Rains and H. D. Ritchie (H. K. Lewis).
Principles of Surgery, S. Schwartz & G. T. Shires (McGraw Hill).

Obstetrics and gynaecology

A Practice of Obstetrics and Gynaecology, G. Chamberlain and J. Dewhurst (Pitman).
Aids to Obstetrics and Gynaecology, G. M. Stirrat (Churchill Livingstone).

Paediatrics

Textbook of Paediatrics, J. O. Forfar and G. C. Arneil (Churchill Livingstone).
Nelson Textbook of Pediatrics, R. E. Behrman and V. C. Vaughan (Saunders).

Psychiatry

Psychiatry, W. H. Trethowan (Baillière Tindall).
Psychiatry for Students, D. Stafford-Clark and A. C. Smith (Allen & Unwin).

The medical course includes many subjects other than those mentioned in the above list, such as the medical and surgical specialties, the organization of medical practice, the public health, the care of the elderly and so on. So far as I know, only one attempt has been made to bring this whole 'knowledge-base' together, a joint effort by the Edinburgh medical school and Blackwell Scientific Publications. The result, in three massive volumes, is *A Companion to Medical Studies*, edited by R. Passmore and J. S. Robson (Blackwell Scientific Publications).

SPECIALIST PUBLICATIONS

Because of the size and no doubt the relative affluence of the market, the qualified doctor is comparatively well served with monographs on particular aspects both of theory and of practice; there is also a very large number of specialist journals, but for the equally important task of keeping up to date with the general progress of medicine, many of us rely a good deal on the weekly journals, which contain short review articles. These include the *British Medical Journal* and *The Lancet* in this country and the *New England Journal of Medicine* and the *Journal of the American Medical Association* in the USA. Computerized 'up-dates' are becoming available, and those available in the USA are regularly reviewed in the *Annals of Internal Medicine*. It would not be possible to review the field of monographs and periodic literature in general, but I will end with a classified list of books chosen either because they relate to particular topics dealt with in the various chapters of this book, or because they have had an important influence on medical thinking.

Genetic disorders

Elements of Medical Genetics, A. E. H. Emery (Churchill Livingstone). A lucid introduction.
Mendelian Inheritance in Man, V. McKusick (McGraw Hill). More advanced treatment.
The Metabolic Basis of Inherited Disease, J. B. Stanbury, J. B. Wyngaarden and D. S. Frederickson (McGraw Hill). Comprehensive textbook of inherited disorders.

Immunology

Clinical Aspects of Immunology, P. J. Lachmann and D. K. Peters (Blackwell Scientific Publications). Comprehensive textbook.

Environment and health

The Role of Medicine – Dream, Mirage, or Nemesis, T. McKeown (Blackwell). This general account of the nature of disease is relevant both to chapter 2, and to the societal aspects treated in chapter 8.
Inequalities in Health, P. Townsend and N. Davidson (Penguin Books). Discussion on the relation between social class and health.
The Health of the Developing World, C. F. Brockington (Book Guild). Contrasts health status in 'developed' and 'developing' countries.
The Diseases of Occupations, Donald Hunter (English University Press). An inspirational textbook of occupational medicine.

Statistics, epidemiology and public health

Invitation to Statistics, G. Kennedy (Blackwell). Introductory, with medical examples.
Principles of Medical Statistics, Sir Austin Bradford Hill

(Lancet). A classic primer for doctors, which has run through many editions.

Uses of Epidemiology, J. N. Morris (Churchill Livingstone). Reveals the relevance of epidemiology to clinical medicine.

More general accounts of the different branches of community medicine are given in two books:

Oxford Textbook of Public Health (4 volumes), W. W. Holland, R. Detels and G. Knox (Oxford University Press).

Preventive and Community Medicine, D. W. Clark and B. MacMahon (Little, Brown).

Communication

Communication in Medicine, C. M. Fletcher (Nuffield Provincial Hospitals Trust).

Sociology

An Introduction to Medical Sociology, D. Tuckett (Tavistock Publications).

Basic Readings in Medical Sociology, D. Tuckett and J. M. Kaufert (Tavistock Publications).

Economics

Principles of Economic Appraisal in Health Care, M. F. Drummond (Oxford University Press).

The Painful Prescription – Rationing Hospital Care, H. J. Aaron and W. B. Schwartz (Brookings Institution).

Ethics

Doctors' Dilemmas: Medical Ethics and Contemporary Science, M. Phillips and J. Dawson (Harvester Press).

A Dictionary of Medical Ethics, A. S. Duncan, G. R. Dunstan and R. B. Welbourn (Darton, Longman, Todd).

Clinical Ethics, A. R. Jonsen, M. Siegler and W. J. Winslade (Macmillan).

Criticisms and alternatives?

The Unmasking of Medicine, Ian Kennedy (Allen & Unwin). A criticism of medical science and medical dominance.

Effectiveness and Efficiency: Random Reflections on Health Services, A. L. Cochrane (Nuffield Provincial Hospitals Trust). A searching interrogation of medical progress.

The Handbook of Complementary Medicine, S. Fulder (Hodder & Stoughton). A guide to the rich variety of alternatives to scientific medicine, from aromatherapy to zen. As Lincoln is reported to have said, 'those who like this sort of thing will find this the sort of thing they like'. But the book itself is a useful guide.

Family practice

The Family Doctor, Sir Ronald Gibson (Allen & Unwin). An inside view, based on long experience, of general medical practice.

Care of the elderly

Practical Geriatric Medicine, A. N. Exton-Smith and M. E. Weksler (Churchill Livingstone). A review of an important 'new' branches of medical care.

Health services

Power and Responsibility in Health Care, W. J. M. Mackenzie (Nuffield Provincial Hospitals Trust). A look at the 'politics' of the NHS by a distinguished political scientist.

The Making of the National Health Service, J. E. Pater (King Edward's Hospital Fund). Historical account by one of the civil servants involved.

History of the British Medical Association, 1932–1981, E. Grey-Turner and F. M. Sutherland (British Medical Association). Gives a professional view of the setting up of the health service.

Professional or Public Health? R. Illsley (Nuffield Provincial Hospitals Trust). Perspective of a medical sociologist.

Public Participation in Health, R. Maxwell and N. Weaver (King Edward's Hospital Fund). Different perceptions of the health service.

American Medicine and the Public Interest, R. Stevens (Yale University Press).

Further Reading

Medical Practice in Modern England. The Impact of Specialization and State Medicine, R. Stevens (Yale University Press).

Many of the topics I have considered rather briefly have been dealt with at some length, with the lay public in mind, in the *Oxford Companion to Medicine*, ed. J. N. Walton, P. B. Beeson and R. Bodley Scott (Oxford University Press, 1986). More personally than would be appropriate for this present book, I have discussed some controversial aspects of science and medical practice in *An Anthology of False Antitheses*, D. Black (Nuffield Provincial Hospitals Trust, 1984).

Glossary

Although useful, a glossary is of its nature a dull thing, so let me try to introduce it with an interesting note. All professions have their private vocabulary, and long-established ones tend to have the longest ones (though recently the sociologists have been catching up with giant strides). At the risk of special pleading, I believe that the medical vocabulary, like the concept of 'a disease', can be defended on grounds of practical use. The single word, generally of classical origin, may seem long, e.g. dys-diadokokinesia, but it often replaces a whole description. Also, classical languages are in fact terse – the Nazis did not gain much when they replaced 'duodenum' by its synonym 'Zwölffingerdarm', especially when they also favoured a return to Gothic script!

In order to keep this glossary within reasonable bounds, I have assumed some familiarity with general scientific vocabulary and I have also limited it to words that appear several times in the text. The terms have usually been explained as they occurred, but this glossary may serve as a reminder. I have not included all the names of diseases which have been used to exemplify points made in the text, so a pocket medical dictionary might be helpful as a back-up to this limited list of definitions.

Anaemia Deficiency of red cells in the blood.

Antibody A globulin, produced by the immune system (q.v.), which reacts with a specific antigen (q.v.) in such a way as generally to neutralize a harmful effect.

Antigen A substance, usually but not necessarily foreign to the body, which stimulates the immune system (q.v.) to react.

Autosomal Refers to genes or chromosomes other than the 'sex chromosomes', X and Y.

Bacterium A micro-organism which may or may not cause disease.

Cancer Collective term for those tumours which are 'malignant', i.e. can spread both locally and/or to distant parts of the body.

Carcinogen A substance that induces tumour formation when the body is exposed to it.

Carrier Someone who harbours an infective agent and is capable of transmitting it to others, but is not himself ill. Also used to denote someone carrying a recessive defective gene (q.v.).

Chromosome A linear aggregation or 'double helix' of DNA (q.v.) within the nucleus of cells; it contains the genes, the units of genetic information.

Coronary arteries The arteries which supply blood to the heart itself. When blocked by clot, the result is coronary thrombosis.

Diagnosis Denotes both the process by which the nature of an illness is discovered and the word or statement which gives the result of that process.

Diabetes A group of diseases characterized by relative inability to use carbohydrate in the tissues.

DNA An acronym for *d*eoxyribo*n*ucleic *a*cid, the versatile chemical substance which transmits the genetic code.

Dominant As applied to genes (q.v.), and opposed to recessive (q.v.), indicates that an effect will be produced even if only one member of a gene-pair is abnormal.

Dyspnoea Literally 'wrong breathing', but combines the ideas of breathlessness and discomfort or actual pain during respiratory movement.

Endocrine system The system of the body which produces a range of chemical messengers (hormones) which can then modulate the activity of other cells, organs and systems.

Endoscopy The use of instruments which enable illumination and inspection of cavities within the body, such as the stomach and large bowel.

Enzyme One of a class of proteins which specifically catalyse (speed up) particular biochemical reactions.

Epidemiology The study of the distribution of disease states within defined populations – see also *incidence* and *prevalence*.

Gene The unit of heredity, made up of DNA, and forming part of a chromosome.

Genetic manipulation A loose term applied to the procedures in which chromosomes are disrupted, some of the genetic material removed, and transferred to other chromosomes.

Histocompatibility antigens (HLA system) These terms relate to a series of antigens on the cell surface, genetically determined, which are 'foreign' to other individuals of the same species, other than identical twins; this system lies at the base of transplant rejection.

Hormone A substance elaborated in an endocrine gland or tissue which exerts an effect on the function of another tissue to which it is carried in the bloodstream, or otherwise gains access.

Immune system The bodily system which reacts to substances recognized as 'foreign' by increasing the numbers and activity of cells which can neutralize the foreign material either by direct cellular attack or by producing antibodies (q.v.).

Incidence The number of cases of a defined illness or other event occurring anew over a specified period in a defined population. Contrast with *prevalence*.

Infection Invasion by disease-producing micro-organisms (bacteria and viruses).

Inflammation A general term for the various local responses of the body to damaging agents, including infection (see chapter 3).

Insulin A hormone produced in the islet cells of the pancreas which assists the use of carbohydrate in the tissues.

Lesion A useful general term applied to an abnormality, commonly a visible one, produced by an agent of disease.

Mendelian Pertaining to 'single-gene' inheritance, as described by the Abbé Mendel.

Metabolism, metabolic The noun and adjective applied to the complex of chemical reactions occurring in the living body – part of the subject matter of biochemistry.

Metastases Secondary deposits of tumour tissue, remote from the primary site.

Monoclonal antibodies Highly specific antibodies (q.v.) produced by cultures of cloned (genetically identical) cells; availability of panels of such antibodies has enabled specific antigens to be more readily and surely identified.

Mutation A fundamental alteration to a gene (q.v.) produced by chemicals or irradiation, leading to change in future offspring.

Oedema Swelling of a part of the body, due to accumulation of fluid between the cells.

Organelle A general term for organized structures within the cell, e.g. nucleus, mitochondria.

Placebo effect An improvement following the administration of a medicine, which is not accounted for by any specific activity of the medicine.

Polygenic A description of that form of inheritance which does not show Mendelian (q.v.) segregation (see chapter 2), but is carried by many genes, producing graded characteristics such as height, intelligence or blood pressure.

Prevalence The number of cases of a disease or event observed at a given point in time. Contrast with *incidence*.

Prognosis The assessment of the outlook in a given situation; also the statement of that outlook.

Recessive Applied to genes (q.v.), and opposed to 'dominant' (q.v.), implying that both members of a gene-pair must be abnormal for an effect to be produced.

Sign A manifestation of disease discovered on examination.

Symptom A manifestation of disease of which the patient is aware and of which he complains.

Syndrome A useful term for a recognizable group of symptoms and signs which may be caused by one or more diseases. Recognition of a syndrome may point directly to a particular disease, or may be a 'half-way house' to diagnosis, by limiting consideration to a smaller group of possibilities.

Toxin A poison produced by bacteria (q.v.) or other organisms.

Tumour A swelling, possibly but not necessarily cancerous.

Valency A measure of the combining power of a chemical element, e.g. *one* atom of carbon combines with *four* atoms of hydrogen, giving carbon a valency of *four*, that of hydrogen being *one*. The high valency of carbon accounts for the great variety of possible organic compounds.

Virus A submicroscopic filterable agent, generally harmful, e.g. the viruses of influenza, poliomyelitis and the common cold.

X-linked Applied to inherited disorders based on an abnormal gene carried on the female (X) chromosome, e.g. haemophilia (see chapter 2).

Specialization within Medicine

As indicated in chapter 1, there are many specialties within the broad divisions of medicine and surgery. To illustrate this, for it would not be possible to be exhaustive, I give here the list of medical specialties recognized in 1986 by the Joint Committee on Higher Medical Training. Some of them are described in chapter 3, and I list these first. For the others, not described there, I give a brief description.

Cardiovascular disease
Endocrinology and diabetes
Gastro-enterology
Haematology
Immunology and allergy
Neurology
Renal disease
Respiratory medicine
Rheumatology

Accident and emergency medicine Deals with urgent medical cases brought to casualty
Clinical pharmacology and therapeutics The study and use of drugs
Communicable diseases Fevers and infections
Community medicine The health care of populations
Dermatology Skin diseases
Genito-urinary medicine Sexually transmitted diseases
Geriatric medicine The treatment of the elderly

Intensive care Treatment of critically ill patients in special units

Medical oncology The medicinal treatment of tumours

Metabolic medicine Diseases of body chemistry and nutrition

Nuclear medicine Application of radioisotopes to investigation and treatment

Occupational medicine Health problems created in the workplace

Rehabilitation medicine Remedial treatments

Tropical medicine

Some of these specialties are represented only in the larger centres or in special hospitals, but in each district hospital there will be physicians competent to see a wide range of medical problems, referred to them by family doctors for diagnosis and treatment. These are specialists in 'general internal medicine'. Similarly, children are cared for by 'paediatricians' at specialist level, some of whom also specialize in one of the system-related specialties given above, and others in the care of the newborn rather than of older children ('neonatal paediatrician').

Index

pregnancy
  fetal health and, 19–20
  termination to avoid genetic
    disease, 16–17, 20, 174
preventive medicine, 168–74,
    190–1
  social class and, 25–6
  value of, 176–7
private health care, 186–7
probability, epidemiology based
    on, 18
profession, medicine as, 3–5
protein, 30
  in blood, 51–2
psychiatry, 206
psychological factors, health
    influenced by, 23–4
psychosomatic illness, 24
public health, 161–74
  failure to integrate individual
    medicine with, 166–8
  improvements in: through
    medical treatment, 192–5
    through preventive
    medicine,
    168–74
  nineteenth-century reforms,
    162–5
  recognition of responsibility
    for, 161–2
Public Health Act (1848), 164,
    165

quality of life, improvements in,
    195
questioning, diagnosis through,
    82–6
Quinlan, Karen, 44

RNA, 30–1, 32
radiation, cancer due to, 70–1
radioactive isotopes, tests with,
    105–6
radiology, 104–6
Ramazzini, Bernardo, 162
randomized controlled trial,
    130–3
reassurance, doctor's ability to
    provide, 146

recessive genes, 12–13, 14, 202
red blood cells, 52
  deficiency of, 97–8
  destruction of, 55–6, 98
reflex actions, 41, 46
Registration of Births and
    Deaths, 1836 Act for, 165
resources, medical, needs in
    relation to, 178–9
respiratory system, 36
Rhesus factor, effect of, 19
rickets, 14
Royal College of Surgeons, 138
rubella, congenital disease and, 19

sample, representative, 158
sanitation improvements, 161,
    164
scar tissue, 64
scientific knowledge, *see*
    knowledge
screening
  biochemical, disadvantages of, 96
  disease prevention through,
    172–4
secrecy, decline in, 142–3, 146
sensory impulses, 46, 47
sex, biological, establishment of,
    99
Sherrington, Sir Charles, 41
sign, distinction between
    symptom and, 81, 202
skills, relative importance of, 7
skin cancer, 70
sleep, drugs inducing, 124
smallpox eradication, 170
smoking
  advice on, 119, 169
  cancer associated with, 67
social class, health inequalities
    associated with, 24–6, 163,
    170
social conditions, improvements
    in, medical improvements in
    relation to, 192–5
social factors, doctors' awareness
    of, 191–2
social history, diagnosis aided by,
    85

Indexed by Ann Barham